Praise for the First Edition

"Don't wait for a swallowing disaster. This book tells you how to keep a swallowing problem from becoming fatal."

—Henry J. Heimlich, M.D.
Author of *Heimlich's Maneuvers*
1984 Recipient of Albert Lasker Public Service Award

"Well written and easy to read. I think this book will be very helpful to dysphagic patients, their families, and all of us who love to eat. I liked it very much."

—Jeri Logemann, Ph.D., CCC-SLP, BCS-S
Ralph and Jean Sundin Professor
Communication Sciences and Disorders
Northwestern University
Evanston, Illinois

"An extremely useful and potentially life-saving book."

—Christiane Northrup, M.D.
Author of *Mother-Daughter Wisdom*:
*Understanding the Crucial Link Between
Mothers, Daughters, and Health*

"Hits just the right audience with just the right information in a digestible form."

—Paul Raia, Ph.D.
Vice President, Clinical Services
Alzheimer's Association
Massachusetts/New Hampshire Chapter

"Empowering for us as advocates for our patients and our family members. An invaluable resource for the lay reader and the health care professional."

—Sheila Bridge CCC-SLP
Associate Professor, C
North Ca

D1516643

"I devoured this book in one sitting. As an 80-year-old man diagnosed 15 years ago with Parkinson's, I felt this book fit me to a T. It gave me much valuable information and I will certainly recommend it to others in my support group."

—K.I., Windsor, California

"What an eye-opener! Who knew a runny nose could actually be a clue to having a life-threatening swallowing problem. Easy-to-read and packed with life-saving knowledge everyone should know. Especially valuable for families and caregivers of elders with dementia, who often develop swallowing problems."

—Jacqueline Marcell
Author of *Elder Rage*
Host of *Coping with Caregiving* Radio Show

"Drs. Sayadi and Herskowitz have shown compassion and responsiveness to an important need of our seniors—safety in swallowing. This book is a treasure."

—Betty Perkins-Carpenter, Ph.D.
President, Senior Fitness Productions, Inc.
Author of *How To Prevent Falls*

"A must-read for seniors and their caregivers. Should be in the library and on the reading list of every senior center in the country!"

—Eric Andersen
CEO and Co-Founder
MySeniorCenter.com

"I didn't know I had a swallowing problem until I read this book."

—Irwin H. Herskowitz, Ph.D.
Professor Emeritus of Biology (Genetics)
Hunter College, City University of New York

"A well-researched, informative guide for those caring for the elderly or the ill. This book will save lives."

—ForeWord Reviews

"For persons with head and neck cancer—for elderly persons in general—this book will help patients and their families understand and deal with swallowing problems."

—Catherine Thibeault, RN, MSN, MPH
Staff Nurse, Milford Regional Medical Center
Milford, Massachusetts

"Swallowing problems are a key part of the rehabilitation process after severe head trauma. *Swallow Safely* will help save lives by giving family members and other caregivers insight into what can go wrong and what to do about it."

—Dixie Fremont-Smith Coskie
Author of *Unthinkable: Tips for Surviving a Child's Traumatic Brain Injury*

"For people affected neurologically by disorders such as Wilson disease or Parkinson disease, swallowing problems are common and often serious. This book provides a much-needed guide for patients and their families or caregivers."

—Carol Terry
Co-Founder, Past President, and Secretary
Wilson Disease Association

"Medica Roya Sayadi et Medicus Joel Herskowitz scripserunt librum de morbo gluttiendi qui est tam astutus tam gravis quam Merckus Libellus – sed multo iocior legere." *

—Marian Sniffen
Joel Herskowitz's Latin Teacher
at University City (MO) High School

* "Drs. Roya Sayadi and Joel Herskowitz have written a book about maladies of swallowing that is as knowing and as serious as the Merck Manual—but much more fun to read."

"This book brings together the science of swallowing and practical guidance for patients and their caregivers."

—Hideh Shad
Roya Sayadi's Science Teacher
at Hadaf High School, Tehran, Iran

SWALLOW SAFELY

How Swallowing Problems Threaten the Elderly and Others

A Caregiver's Guide to Dysphagia: Recognition, Treatment, and Prevention

Second Edition

Roya Sayadi, Ph.D., CCC-SLP

and

Joel Herskowitz, M.D.

INSIDE/OUTSIDE PRESS

Organizations and businesses that deal with elderly persons and
those with particular medical or neurologic disorders are
invited to contact the publisher for information
as to discounts for bulk purchases.

Inside/Outside Press
11 Wilson Street
Natick, Massachusetts 01760
www.swallowsafely.com
swallowsafely@aol.com

Cover design by Mike Powless of OLM Designs and
Julio Pompa Frizza of Monkey C Media.

Book design by Arrow Graphics, Inc.
info@arrow1.com

Publisher's Cataloging-in-Publication
(Provided by Quality Books, Inc.)

Sayadi, Roya.
    Swallow safely : how swallowing problems threaten the
elderly and others : a caregiver's guide to dysphagia: recognition,
treatment, and prevention / Roya Sayadi and Joel Herskowitz.
    p. cm.
    Includes bibliographical references and index.
    "Help for persons with stroke, Parkinson disease,
multiple sclerosis, Alzheimer disease, ALS, cancer, COPD,
heart disease, and head injury."
    ISBN-13: 978-09819601-5-9

    1. Deglutition disorders–Popular works. 2. Older
people–Care. I. Herskowitz, Joel. II. Title.

RC815.2.S39 2009   616.3'23
                 QBI09-200033

NOTE TO THE READER

This book is intended to provide information for those who wish to learn more about swallowing, related problems, prevention, and treatment. It is in no way intended to replace or to be a substitute for the judgment of a personal treating physician, speech-language pathologist, or other specialist for the diagnosis, treatment, or ongoing care of a patient who has or might have a swallowing problem. The information and opinions provided in this book are believed to be accurate and sound. The reader should consult his or her treating professionals before adopting any of the suggestions in this book.

Recognizing different approaches to the emergency treatment of the conscious choking adult, the publisher and the authors have presented—by means of text and illustrations—principles and practices we believe are consistent with the highest standards of emergency care. For definitive, up-to-the-minute instruction, the reader is referred to the American Heart Association, the American Red Cross, or a certified CPR instructor.

Neither the publisher nor the authors shall have liability or responsibility to any person or entity with respect to any loss, damage, or injury caused, or alleged to have been caused, directly or indirectly, by the use or application of any of the material contained in this book.

Dedication

To Sri Sri Ravi Shankar

Bringing the People of the World
Together in Peace, Health, and Happiness

CONTENTS

ILLUSTRATIONS

SUMMARIES

ABOUT THE AUTHORS

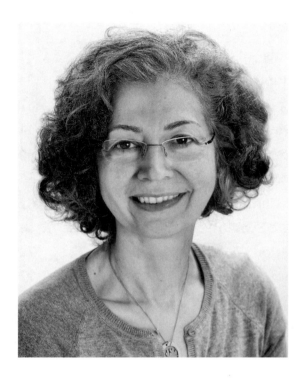

Roya Sayadi, Ph.D., CCC-SLP, is a graduate of the Iran University of Medical Sciences in Tehran. She received her Ph.D. in neurogenic communication disorders from Michigan State University. She has taught speech-language-swallowing pathology at the undergraduate and graduate school levels. She has extensive clinical experience working with persons who have swallowing problems associated with a wide variety of medical and neurologic illnesses. She lives in Natick, Mass., with her husband. They have four children.

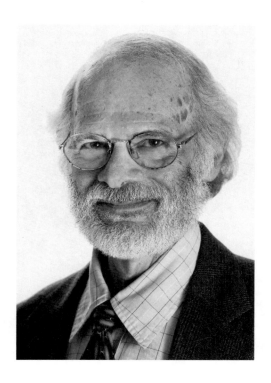

Joel Herskowitz, M.D., Dr. Sayadi's husband, is a graduate of Princeton University and the Albert Einstein College of Medicine. A board-certified pediatric neurologist, he is on the faculty of the Boston University School of Medicine. He is the author of *Pediatrics, Neurology, and Psychiatry: Common Ground* (with N. Paul Rosman, M.D.), *Is Your Child Depressed?*, and *TWISTED!*, a play about a woman with Wilson disease, which he has presented in Boston, Chicago, St. Louis, and Heidelberg, Germany.

Photographs by John Mottern

ACKNOWLEDGMENTS

As a student of speech-language pathology, everything I learned about swallowing I learned from Jeri Logemann. A professor at Northwestern University and its School of Medicine, Dr. Logemann is a towering figure and pioneer in the field of speech-language pathology. I came under her influence through her classic textbook, *Evaluation and Treatment of Swallowing Disorders*, as a graduate student, through periodicals she edited, through conferences I was privileged to attend, and through conversations I had with her in person. We have been honored by her endorsement of the first edition of this book and are saddened to learn of her passing in June of 2014. (R.S.)

We thank my parents, Irwin H. Herskowitz, Ph.D., and Reida Postrel Herskowitz, both of whom are now deceased, for their critical and helpful reviews of earlier printings; Barrie S. Greiff, M.D., author, psychiatrist, and friend, for his encouragement and suggestions; Henry J. Heimlich, M.D., for his review of portions of the first edition; the late Anet James for her superb illustrations; John Mottern for his photographic contributions; and my sister, Mara Herskowitz, for the cover photograph. (J.H.)

Lastly, we acknowledge the contribution of Jamie McDonough, a young man who, in bravely facing the challenges of Wilson disease, made us feel that this book can serve a real purpose—not just for the ill, frail, and elderly—but *for persons of any age* whose neurologic disorder or medical condition affects their swallowing and puts them at risk.

Roya Sayadi and Joel Herskowitz
Natick, Massachusetts
July 2016

CHAPTER 1

WHY WE WROTE THIS BOOK

WHY WE WROTE
THIS BOOK

M any people these days know about the dangers of falling in the elderly. A hip fracture, a head injury—a funeral. Falls account for some 30,000 deaths per year in this country.

Doctors stress fall prevention. Magazine articles and books are devoted to the subject. Caregivers are on the alert.

You do many things to reduce the risk of falling in an ill or frail loved one. You watch out for medications that can cause lightheadedness or drowsiness, provide for proper nutrition and hydration, promote strength and balance through exercise, get rid of throw rugs that can slip, keep living spaces well lit, provide handholds in the bathroom, and work with your doctor in monitoring your loved one for infectious illness.

The payoff is greater safety, independence, and peace of mind—theirs and yours.

Swallowing Problems: Another Major Concern

Did you know that *swallowing problems* are another major threat to the ill or frail elderly? They, too, account for tens of thousands of deaths in the United States every year. More, it appears, than falls.

The United States Agency for Healthcare Research and Quality has estimated that 60,000 Americans die each year from complications associated with swallowing problems.

- **Choking** takes nearly four thousand lives.

- **Aspiration** of food, liquid, medication, or saliva loaded with bacteria into the lungs causes fatal pneumonia in tens of thousands.

- **Malnutrition** resulting from swallowing problems causes weakness and susceptibility to infection that hasten the death of thousands more.

- **Dehydration** associated with swallowing impairment contributes to falls, strokes, and other causes of premature death.

A Vulnerable Population: The Ill and The Frail

Nearly 40 million Americans in a total U.S. population of just over 300 million are elderly (65 years of age and older). *From 15 to 50 percent of the elderly are estimated to have a swallowing problem.* That's somewhere between six and 20 million people—and the number is growing.

Swallowing problems account for billions of dollars annually as a result of diagnostic tests, hospitalization, and aftercare costs such as rehabilitation centers, nursing homes, and home-care services. That does not include out-of-pocket and work-related expenses incurred by families involved in caregiving—not to mention the incalculable emotional toll.

So, in terms of lives lost, dollars spent, and schedules disrupted, swallowing problems are no small matter. They are huge.

Has This Happened To You?

When you sit down to dinner with your mother, do you wonder why she constantly clears her throat?

Do you ever ask yourself why her nose runs while eating?

When you give your father juice, do you hold your breath waiting to see if it goes down the right tube?

When he eats a sandwich, are you on the edge of your seat fearing you'll need to perform the Heimlich maneuver?

Are you forever looking at the kitchen clock when you eat with your mother because meals take so long?

Does your loved one sometimes feel light-headed or faint with swallowing?

Do you wonder how your loved one can possibly be getting enough food or liquid to survive?

If you've had any of these concerns, you may be facing significant swallowing issues.

How This Book Came About

This book came about because Roya, a speech-language pathologist practicing in the Greater Boston Area, was seeing patient after patient with swallowing problems.

These patients—not all elderly—had a wide variety of medical and neurologic disorders: stroke, Parkinson disease, congestive heart failure, cancer, diabetes, kidney disease, COPD (chronic obstructive pulmonary disease), multiple sclerosis, ALS (Lou Gehrig's disease), diabetes, head injury, and Alzheimer disease among others.

They all had swallowing problems!

Typical Scenarios

A 62-year-old man with ***Parkinson disease*** did everything slowly. Not only were his arms and legs involved, his tongue was, too. So he had difficulty chewing, moving food along, and finally swallowing. Food often got stuck in his throat and caused him to cough and gag.

A 50-year-old woman with a recent ***stroke*** had difficulty drinking liquids compared with swallowing solid foods. Liquids rushed ahead to cause fits of coughing that brought tears to her eyes. A bout of pneumonia put her back into the hospital and delayed her neurologic recovery.

An 82-year-old man with *Alzheimer disease* who loved ice cream required continuous assistance with feeding. He was extremely distractible and could no longer use a fork or spoon. He had also "forgotten" what to do with food once it was in his mouth. A single swallow could take three minutes or longer. He was always on the verge of dehydration, which would increase his risk of falling.

A 56-year-old woman treated for *salivary gland cancer* had an extremely dry mouth and exquisitely painful sores inside her cheeks. Chewing was painful and her lack of saliva made it difficult to "glue together" a ball of food suitable for swallowing. Eating was an unpleasant experience that left her physically and emotionally drained.

A 42-year-old man with *multiple sclerosis* was able to chew. But when it came to the actual swallow, some of the food was left behind in his throat. It got sucked into his airway; and, because his cough was so weak, he could not expel the material. So it made its way to his lungs to cause pneumonia.

A typical patient of Roya's had more than one health condition. Parkinson disease, COPD, heart disease, and diabetes in the same person would not be unusual. Also typical would be for a patient to be taking a dozen medications every day. Their side effects—most notably dry mouth—sometimes caused or contributed to swallowing difficulty.

When these patients (or their caregivers) understood the nature of the swallowing problem—especially how it might threaten survival or quality of life—they were better able to follow treatment recommendations and advocate more strongly for themselves.

Knowledge Can Be Life-Saving

Recognizing this knowledge gap, we wanted to write a book that would educate and empower patients and their caregivers.

We have written this book to

- give you a basic understanding of swallowing
- show you how things can go wrong
- explain why swallowing problems such as choking and aspiration are serious
- tell you how to recognize swallowing problems before they become life-threatening pneumonia, malnutrition, or dehydration
- explain how medications can cause or complicate swallowing problems
- touch upon end-of-life issues related to swallowing and
- guide you as to how to organize your observations, questions, and concerns in getting help for yourself or a loved one.

This book is not intended to be an exhaustive treatment of swallowing problems. Nor is it intended to be a substitute for hands-on evaluation, diagnosis, and treatment by a physician or speech-language pathologist.

Our **References** and **Additional Readings** will allow you to read further in areas of interest. Our **Resources** section can put you in touch with others who share your concerns and can be of help.

Choking: A Much-Feared Problem

Choking can cause a tremendous amount of anxiety in a patient or caregiver. We devote an entire chapter to choking. We define *choking* and explain how it occurs. We discuss who is at increased risk of choking and how you can reduce this risk. We explain what to do if your loved one—or you—choke.

Crucial Decisions

Because swallowing is vital to nutrition and health, it often becomes a focal point in quality-of-life and end-of-life issues. We feel that our book can help patients and their families in making difficult decisions by giving them a better understanding of swallowing problems and treatment options.

Having cared for close family members with swallowing problems related to stroke and cancer, we have experienced first-hand some of the challenges you may be facing.

What's Your Swallowing Story?

We have been struck that almost everyone we meet has a swallowing story. People tell us about an elderly aunt who feared that choking, not cancer, would kill her.

They also tell us how they were eating carelessly at a banquet and found themselves on the receiving end of a Heimlich maneuver that saved their life.

Swallow Safely At Any Age

It's not just the elderly who are at risk of swallowing problems. Any adult with medical or neurologic illness—such as lung disease, congestive heart failure, head and neck cancer, stroke, multiple sclerosis, ALS, Guillain-Barré syndrome, or Parkinson disease—is vulnerable and will find our discussion of swallowing and its disorders relevant.

We hope, too, that this book will make *you* more mindful of your own swallowing and prevent problems that could cost you your life.

And don't forget about your children. Help them establish healthy swallowing habits so that eating and drinking are pleasurable and safe.

Roya's patients and their families tell her: "We didn't realize there was so much to swallowing. We wish we'd known about this sooner."

Joel's father said: "I didn't know I had a swallowing problem until I read this book."

We believe this book will provide you with useful, potentially life-saving information. We wish you the best in helping special persons in your life to **SWALLOW SAFELY.**

CHAPTER 2

HOW SWALLOWING WORKS

HOW SWALLOWING WORKS

Before we look at how things can go wrong, let's look briefly at normal swallowing. The purpose of swallowing is to bring food, liquid, or medication safely from the mouth to the stomach.

Keep in mind that swallowing does not occur in isolation. Throughout the process, signals are sent continuously to and from the nervous system to coordinate swallowing with breathing.

Swallowing is more than a one-step gulp-and-gone. It's a process. You can use the word **"POPE"** to remember its four phases:

- **Preparatory**
- **Oral**
- **Pharyngeal**
- **Esophageal**

1. Preparatory Phase—Forming a Ball of Food

The Preparatory Phase begins even before food gets to your mouth. Your sense of smell—even the anticipation of food—can make your mouth water.

When you take a bite of food, a remarkable dance begins. Your jaws, teeth, cheeks, and tongue work together to make the food into more or less of a ball.

This ball of food is called a *bolus* after the Latin word for "lump."

Your lips close tightly so food doesn't escape from your mouth. Your teeth (or dentures) grind the food into smaller bits. Saliva flows from under and around your tongue. It moistens the food, gathering with it flaky food bits or nearby sugar particles (see Fig. 2-1).

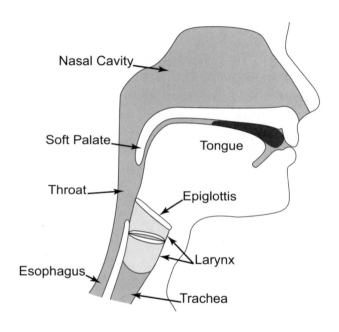

Figure 2-1: Preparatory Phase. Jaws and tongue reduce food to a pasty bolus (in black). (Adapted with permission from *Evaluation and Treatment of Swallowing Disorders, 2nd Ed.*, p. 28, by J.A. Logemann. Copyright 1998 by PRO-ED, Inc., Austin, TX.)

Your tongue mixes and churns the food. It directs the bolus to one side then the other, where your teeth grind it into a dough-like paste. Your jaws move not only up-and-down but in a rotary manner that maximizes grinding.

In addition to physically reducing the mass of solid food, chewing enhances flavor. Juices and other flavorful food elements leak out to contact your taste buds. Enzymes in saliva get to work right away. They start to break down the food while it's still in your mouth.

Your sense of smell gets into the act once again. Aromas pass from throat to nasal cavity where smell receptors enhance the taste of the food and stimulate further saliva flow.

Coordination Required. Just as skilled dancers don't step on each other's toes, we (usually) do not chew on our tongue.

Why not? The tongue sends continuous signals to the brain telling it where the tongue is and what it's doing. Your gums, cheeks, lips, and palate also send information to the brain so you can chew without worrying about chomping on your tongue.

Likewise, breathing and swallowing must work closely together for swallowing to be safe.

Ordinarily, breathing can continue during the Preparatory Phase. But when a medical or neurologic disorder interferes with the balance between the two, breathing and swallowing can become dangerously out of synch.

And, if—under any circumstance—you stir things up by attempting to swallow while distracted, talking, chewing, laughing, *and* breathing, you're asking for trouble. (See Chapters 4 and 5, which discuss *choking* and *aspiration*.)

2. Oral Phase—Transport From Mouth to Throat

Your tongue is now loaded with food. It's like a bucket without a handle. The tongue squeezes the ball of food against the hard palate. This carries the bolus from the front to the back of the mouth, where the *pharynx*, or *throat*, begins.

When you open your mouth in front of a mirror, the very back part of what you see is your *throat*. Actually it is the oral portion of the pharynx, the *oropharynx*. Just above is the *nasopharynx* and below is the *hypopharynx* (see Fig. 2-2).

The exquisite coordination seen in the Preparatory Phase continues.

- Your lips remain closed to prevent food or liquid from escaping from the front of your mouth.
- Your cheeks stiffen and press against your gums and teeth, which keeps food from falling into pockets between cheek and gum.

- Your tongue presses against the bony roof of your mouth to form a muscular chute that directs food to the throat.
- These structures work together during the Oral Phase to generate air pressure that moves the bolus along.

The entire Oral Phase generally takes about one second.

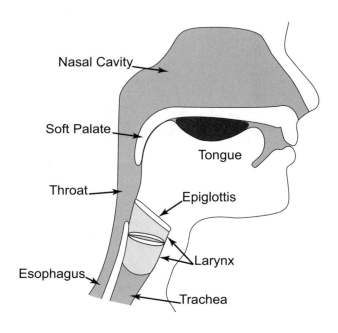

Figure 2-2: Oral Phase. The bolus (in black) is brought from the front to the back of the mouth. (Adapted with permission from *Evaluation and Treatment of Swallowing Disorders, 2nd Ed.*, p. 28, by J.A. Logemann. Copyright 1998 by PRO-ED, Inc., Austin, TX.)

3. Pharyngeal Phase—Pushing It Down

The Pharyngeal Phase includes the *swallowing reflex*. It is activated automatically by food, liquid (including saliva), or medication reaching the pharynx (see Fig. 2-3). Its entrance is marked by the fleshy pillars that frame the tonsils.

This reflex, mediated through the brainstem, coordinates the many muscles required to push the food down into the esophagus while acting as a safety net to keep it from going where it does not belong: the respiratory tract.

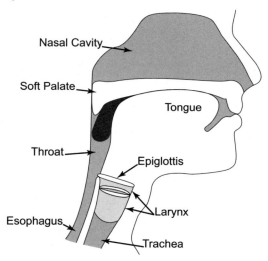

Figure 2-3: Pharyngeal Phase. The bolus (in black) reaches the pharynx to trigger the swallowing reflex. Note the protective changes in position of the soft palate and the epiglottis. (Adapted with permission from *Evaluation and Treatment of Swallowing Disorders, 2nd Ed.*, p. 28, by J.A. Logemann. Copyright 1998 by PRO-ED, Inc., Austin, TX.)

Six hundred or so swallows a day. That's a big job. Without conscious direction, the swallowing reflex weaves together many elements so you can swallow safely.

Here's what happens during the Pharyngeal Phase:

1. Breathing stops briefly.

2. The tongue and soft palate seal off the roof of the mouth so food doesn't escape through the nose.

3. The hinge-like epiglottis closes over the entrance to the larynx (voice box), which helps keep food, liquid, or pills from entering the airway.

4. The larynx moves forward and upward, opening the upper esophagus and further preventing food from getting to the lungs.

5. Within the larynx, the vocal cords come together to keep food or liquid from entering the trachea (windpipe).

6. Muscles of the pharynx and tongue contract to move the bolus to and through the upper part of the esophagus.

7. The *upper esophageal sphincter (UES)*, a ring-shaped muscle at the uppermost esophagus, relaxes to allow food to pass from throat to esophagus (see Fig. 2-4).

Because many different foods and liquids of different amounts and textures pass from your mouth to your stomach, it will come as no surprise that your swallowing apparatus is constantly adjusting to these ever-changing demands for safe swallowing.

The entire Pharyngeal Phase normally takes a second or less. Breathing resumes after the swallow.

A word or two about *gagging* and *vomiting*. While the swallowing reflex invites food *in*, gagging and

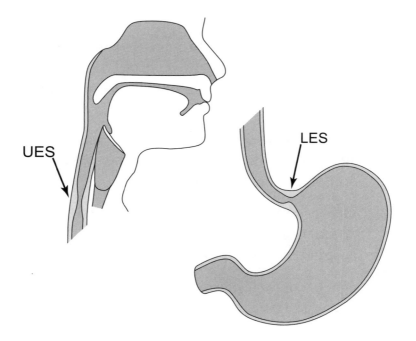

Figure 2-4: Esophageal Sphincters. Food enters the esophagus through the upper esophageal sphincter (UES) and enters the stomach through the lower esophageal sphincter (LES).

vomiting reflexively send material *out*. A brisk gag does *not* mean a person has a normal swallow. And, as we will discuss in a later chapter, *gagging* does not mean *choking*.

4. Esophageal Phase—Getting to the Stomach

Once the bolus gets past the upper esophageal sphincter (UES), this muscular structure contracts tightly to guard against backflow (see Figs. 2-4 and 2-5).

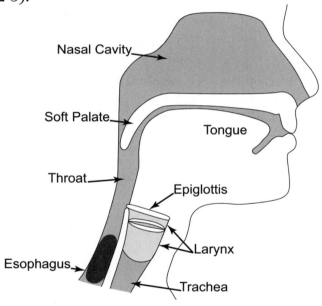

Figure 2-5: Esophageal Phase. The bolus (in black) leaves the pharynx en route to the stomach. (Adapted with permission from *Evaluation and Treatment of Swallowing Disorders, 2nd Ed.*, p. 28, by J.A. Logemann. Copyright 1998 by PRO-ED, Inc., Austin, TX.)

The bolus works its way through the esophagus, moved along by orderly waves of contraction (called *peristalsis*) to reach the *lower esophageal sphincter* (LES) (see Fig. 2-4). Like its upper counterpart, the lower esophageal sphincter is contracted (closed) at rest. So it must relax to let food pass into the stomach. The entire trip through the esophagus normally takes from eight to twenty seconds.

Phases of Swallowing

1. Preparatory	Forming a ball of food
2. Oral	Bringing it from mouth to throat
3. Pharyngeal	Pushing the food down safely
4. Esophageal	Getting food to the stomach

Putting It All Together

Let's go for a swallowing walk-through. Tear off a piece of warm, crusty, freshly-baked bread. Hold it in front of you and look at it. Your nose picks up the pleasant smell and saliva flows as you prepare for food to enter your mouth.

The bread passes your lips, and you bite off a hunk. Your tongue greets it and mixes it with saliva, forming a ball of food as it gathers up bits of flaky crust so you don't inhale them. It moves the food to the side where your teeth begin to chew.

Your jaws move up and down, side to side. This rotary action grinds the food until it becomes pasty. You continue to breathe while you chew. Your tongue gathers the bolus into a central valley in your mouth, then presses it against the bony palate. Your lips continue their tight seal and your cheeks stiffen further, pressing against your teeth and gums.

The food is brought to the back of your mouth where muscles of the throat and palate block escape through your nose. The bolus enters the pharynx. Now comes the moment of truth—the swallow itself.

Like a track athlete getting ready for a jump, you pause, gather energy, and hold your breath. Your tongue and throat muscles forcefully contract. Your Adam's apple rises as your larynx elevates and squeezes tightly shut, closing off the airway. You swallow. The food leaves your throat and begins its downward descent. You release air through your nose as you resume breathing.

Your tongue searches out remnants of food that may have been left behind between gum and cheek or stuck to the roof of your mouth. You swallow one or several times more to finish things off, perhaps clearing your throat between swallows. The final swallow is little more than saliva.

You can turn this thought exercise into a real-life experience by getting a piece of bread or chunk of apple and observing yourself as you chew and swallow.

See if you can follow the various phases. Notice especially how many roles the tongue plays. Making food into a ball. Positioning it for chewing. Bringing it to the back of the mouth. Pushing against the hard palate and down. Cleaning up afterwards. Did you notice how breathing stops during the swallow itself?

We think you'll agree—there's a lot going on here. Swallowing is a complicated process, something we generally take for granted when all is well.

But all is not always well. In the next chapter, keeping the phases of swallowing in mind, we look at how swallowing can break down.

CHAPTER 3

WHEN SWALLOWING
DOESN'T WORK

WHEN SWALLOWING DOESN'T WORK

Now that we've looked at normal swallowing phase by phase, you have a framework for understanding how things can go wrong.

Before going any further, we need to introduce an important word: *dysphagia* (pronounced "diss-FAY-juh"). Simply put, dysphagia means "difficulty swallowing." (Note: *dysphagia* should not be confused with *dysphasia*, a disorder of language.)

Difficulty swallowing is *always* of concern. It can put a person at risk of choking and aspiration, interfere with proper nutrition and hydration, and make meals anxiety-provoking, time-consuming, and frustrating.

What Dysphagia Feels Like

These are some of the things people complain of when they have difficulty swallowing:

"The food doesn't go down."

"I have to swallow more than once."

"Tears come to my eyes when I eat."

"My nose runs at mealtimes."

"Pills get stuck in my throat."

"I cough when I drink water."

"The food falls out of my mouth."

"I have a hard time eating steak."

"When I swallow, juice goes up my nose."

"It hurts when I swallow."

"I get hiccups a lot."

"I'm afraid I'm going to choke."

"My voice sounds funny after I eat."

"I'm always burping."

"I get so tired, I can't finish a meal."

"What do you expect? I'm old."

Sometimes a person has no complaint at all—but a serious swallowing problem nonetheless. (This occurs with *silent aspiration*. See Chapter 5.)

Where Swallowing Breaks Down

Swallowing problems can arise at any step in the swallowing process (Fig. 3-1). They can result from structural, neurologic, medical, or psychologic causes.

Structural refers to anatomy. Something is missing (due to birth defect, injury, or surgery) or extra (such as a cancerous growth, cyst, diverticulum, or aneurysm).

Neurologic refers to a disease process involving the nervous system that interferes with muscle control, speed, or coordination (as with Parkinson disease, stroke, multiple sclerosis, ALS, Guillain-Barré syndrome, or diphtheria).

Medical refers to a condition that causes overall weakness (such as congestive heart failure) or breathing difficulty (such as COPD).

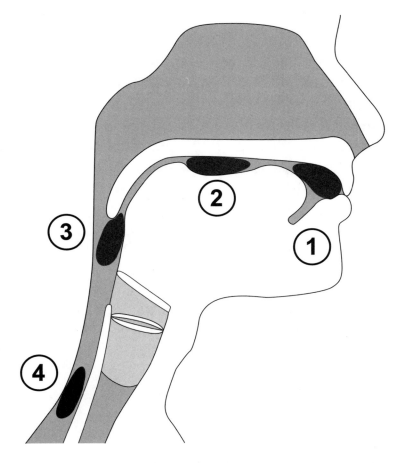

Figure 3-1: Four Phases of Normal Swallowing.
(1) Preparatory, (2) Oral, (3) Pharyngeal, (4) Esophageal.

Swallowing and Aging

Not surprisingly, as we grow older, our swallowing slows down. This is not generally a problem. But combining age-related medical or neurologic conditions with the effects of medication increases the risk of a swallowing problem.

Dangerous Circumstances

Even if you don't have a structural, neurologic, or medical problem, swallowing can break down. This can happen at your own dinner table when you're eating and talking, at a noisy school cafeteria when children rush through a too-short lunch period to get to the playground for a few cherished minutes, or at a bar when you're drinking alcohol and having a good time laughing it up with friends.

A person of any age who participates in a food-eating contest—involving such items as hot dogs, hard-boiled eggs, cupcakes, sausage, or gulab jamuns (an Indian sweet about the size of a "donut hole")—is putting himself in harm's way. (These examples are based upon real-life death reports.)

1. Preparatory Phase Problems

As we have seen, a good supply of saliva helps to make a well-chewed, pasty bolus that slides safely through the mouth, throat, and esophagus. Saliva binds the various foodstuffs to form a cohesive bolus.

Cut down on your saliva flow (through dehydration, drug effect, or diseases such as Sjögren's syndrome) and you can interfere with any phase of swallowing. This can be the tipping point for a serious swallowing problem.

Losing one's sense of smell or taste can also reduce the supply of saliva. This can result from infections of the nose, mouth, or throat; tobacco use; allergies; dental disease; diabetes; underactive thyroid; medication (see Chapter 6); Parkinson disease; Alzheimer disease; Huntington disease; multiple sclerosis; brain tumor; vitamin or mineral deficiency (including B12 or zinc); radiotherapy; chemotherapy; or Sjögren's syndrome.

Keep in mind that anything blocking the sense of smell will also interfere with taste sensation. Furthermore, a medication might not *abolish* the sense of taste but *alter* it, for example, making a food taste "metallic."

Swallowing and Dehydration. Dehydration is caused by too little water coming in, too much water going out, or both. A person who is dehydrated will urinate less often, produce less saliva, and often be constipated. He or she will be at increased risk of infection such as UTI or pneumonia.

It's not just swallowing that suffers when you're dehydrated. Dehydration also means less blood to the brain and muscles. That can interfere with thinking, balance, and overall strength—making a person confused, dizzy, weak, and additionally vulnerable

Causes of Dehydration

- Lack of thirst commonly occurs with Alzheimer disease, stroke, brain tumor, head trauma, and old age.

- Some people might avoid going to the kitchen or bathroom for a drink of water because weakness, dizziness, or loss of balance makes it difficult or dangerous to do so.

- Neurologic disorders such as Parkinson disease, multiple sclerosis, Alzheimer disease, ALS, and stroke can slow down eating and drinking to such a degree that it becomes impossible to take in adequate food or liquid by mouth. This is also true for persons with an exquisitely sore mouth and throat due to cancer treatment.

- Depressed persons often lose their appetite for liquids as well as for food. Antidepressant medication can make matters worse by causing dry mouth (see Chapter 6).

- Excessive water loss from sweating may result from environmental causes. The thermostat is set too high. The air conditioner is not working. A person is under too many blankets.

- The nearly continuous muscle activity that can occur with dystonia, Wilson disease, and some forms of cerebral palsy can similarly cause significant water loss due to sweating.

- Increased urination with *diabetes mellitus* ("sugar diabetes"), *diabetes insipidus* (following head trauma or with renal disease), or *diuretic medication* (used to treat congestive heart failure or high blood pressure) can lead to dehydration.

- Vomiting, diarrhea, or fever can cause dehydration as well.

to falling. Plus, being dehydrated can make you feel just plain miserable—even depressed.

Effects of Cancer Treatment. Radiotherapy or chemotherapy can cause dry mouth (*xerostomia*, pronounced "ZERO-stoe-mee-uh") and cracking of mucous membranes that line the mouth and throat. They can also interfere with a person's immune system, setting the stage for infection with yeast or other germs.

As a result, movements of the lip, cheek, or tongue can become exquisitely painful. This can make chewing and swallowing extremely unpleasant, creating a vicious cycle of dehydration, malnutrition, and weakness—leading to more of the same.

Denture Danger. Poorly fitting dentures—often associated with painful gums—can interfere with chewing and pave the way for major problems. Add impatience, inattentiveness, difficulty cutting with a knife and fork, and a bit of alcohol and you have a recipe for a choking emergency (see Chapter 4).

Dentures (and underlying gums) that are not cleaned regularly are a rich source of bacteria that can get to the lungs to cause pneumonia (see *Oral Care Counts* in Chapter 8).

Pulmonary Problems. For a mouth-breather the simple act of swallowing can be a disaster waiting to happen. A poorly timed, gasping breath by a person with COPD can suck food, liquid, or medication into the lungs (*aspiration*) to cause pneumonia. Or the airway can get blocked (*choking*), presenting an immediate threat to life.

Drinking from a cup can be a particular challenge for persons with respiratory disease. When we drink, we usually take a series of gulps while holding our breath for several seconds. That brief period without breathing may be more than someone with respiratory illness can tolerate. It can lead to gasping and anxiety that make swallowing unsafe.

2. Oral Phase Problems

The Oral Phase is all about transport. Having a dry mouth interferes not just with bolus formation but also with passage of the bolus through the mouth.

As you know, the tongue plays the key role in bringing food from the front to the back of the mouth, where the swallowing reflex takes over. Anything that affects the structure or function of the tongue will influence swallowing, for example, surgical removal of part of the tongue in treating cancer.

With neurologic disorders such as Parkinson disease, brainstem stroke, Guillain-Barré syndrome, ALS, Wilson disease, and Huntington disease, slow, poorly controlled tongue, lip, and jaw movements interfere with bolus formation and transport. Dehydration, malnutrition, and the threat of choking or aspiration are constant concerns.

The Tongue's Many Roles

Promotes taste and enjoyment of food

Places food in position for chewing

Mixes food with saliva to create bolus

Transports bolus from front to back of mouth

Helps push food down

Cleans up after the swallow

Swallowing and Stroke. Swallowing problems are a common, potentially life-threatening complication of stroke. They account for thousands of deaths per year. The type of swallowing problem depends upon the nature and extent of the stroke: hemispheric or brainstem, motor or sensory.

The good news is that through effective medical care and specific swallowing therapy many persons who have suffered a stroke will survive and be able to safely resume eating a relatively normal diet within weeks to months.

Paralysis or weakness of tongue, lip, or cheek muscles can interfere with chewing, transport, swallowing, and cleaning up after the swallow. Food spills out from the front of the mouth. Liquids get to the throat without control or direction before protective mechanisms (including cough) can be called into play. Food left behind can readily be aspirated.

Loss of Sensation. Sensory loss, too, can throw off any phase of swallowing. The brain needs to know what kind of food the mouth is working on, where the bolus is, and whether any food remains after the swallow. When sensation is absent, the swallowing reflex will not be triggered.

Loss of sensation (affecting mouth, throat, or larynx) can also interfere with coughing. Without an effective cough response, food, liquid (including saliva), or medication that gets into the airway is more likely to reach the lungs.

3. Pharyngeal Phase Problems

Food reaching the pharynx activates the swallowing reflex. As we saw in Chapter 2, many things come together to make swallowing safe.

The swallowing reflex is based in the brainstem, the lowermost part of the brain (between the cerebrum and the spinal cord). Neurologic disorders affecting this part of the nervous system will influence the Pharyngeal Phase of swallowing. These disorders include multiple sclerosis, Parkinson disease, ALS, Guillain-Barré syndrome, and some types of stroke.

Voice Problems. Voice problems are of serious concern and call for prompt medical examination. They are often associated with swallowing problems, especially those that involve the pharyngeal phase. Because the larynx (the *voice* box) is the last level of protection for the airway, anything that interferes with its working properly can increase the risk of aspiration and choking.

A *nasal quality* to the voice or regurgitation of liquid through the nose suggests inadequate closure of the soft palate, a hallmark of ALS and diphtheria.

A *hoarse voice* resulting from paralysis of the recurrent laryngeal nerve, suggests inadequate closure of the vocal cords, thereby allowing ready aspiration. This can result from lung cancer, pulmonary tuberculosis, or accidentally during surgery among other causes.

A *weak voice*—as with myasthenia gravis, muscular dystrophy, or multiple sclerosis—can be associated with swallowing problems because the muscles are too weak to push the food down. Overall weakness due to heart disease, lung problems, or cancer can have the same effect.

A weak, *monotone voice* with imprecise articulation is a hallmark of Parkinson disease. With Parkinson disease significant swallowing problems can occur at any phase of swallowing: preparatory, oral, pharyngeal, or esophageal.

Intubation and Swallowing Problems. Persons who have undergone intubation—placement of a tube into the trachea to support breathing—can later experience swallowing difficulties. Scar tissue resulting from difficult or prolonged intubation can prevent complete closure of the vocal cords during the swallowing reflex, thereby increasing the risk of aspiration.

Zenker Diverticulum. Swallowing is a muscular activity. It generates great force within the throat. Not surprisingly, decades of swallowing can weaken the pharynx and cause throat tissue to balloon out or protrude.

Such an outpouching, called a *Zenker diverticulum*, commonly forms where the throat meets the esophagus. As a result, food can get trapped en route to the stomach and hide out in this pouch. That can lead to bad breath, frequent coughing, regurgitation, or worse—choking or aspiration.

4. Esophageal Phase Problems

After passing through the pharynx, the bolus reaches the esophagus. It enters the esophagus through the upper esophageal sphincter (UES) (see Fig. 2-4).

Recall that this sphincter, a ring-like muscle, is usually contracted and relaxes as part of the swallowing reflex to let food pass through.

With neurologic disorders, formation of scar tissue, or compression by a tumor within the chest (for example, a thyroid cancer), the UES may not open fully. As a result, the entire bolus cannot get to the esophagus. This leaves residue in the throat, from which it can be readily aspirated.

If the upper esophageal sphincter shuts too soon, it can pinch off part of the bolus before it enters the esophagus. In either case, food stays in the throat, ready to fall (or be inhaled) into an unprotected airway.

Achalasia: A Failure To Relax. The lower esophageal sphincter is the gateway to the stomach (see Fig. 2-4). With *achalasia* ("ay-kuh-LAY-zhuh"), this sphincter fails to relax to permit the bolus to enter the stomach.

This creates a backup much like a clogged drainpipe. Persons with achalasia may have difficulty swallowing, a feeling of fullness, chest discomfort, or regurgitation.

Other Esophageal Problems. The esophagus is a favorite target of *scleroderma*, an autoimmune disorder that affects connective tissue. Stiffened esophageal walls or constricting scar tissue can interfere with passage of a bolus. Achalasia and *esophagitis*—inflammation of the esophagus—also commonly occur with scleroderma.

Eosinophilic esophagitis is marked by infiltration of the esophageal lining (its *mucosa*) by eosinophils, a type of white blood cell typically associated with allergic conditions.

With *gastroesophageal reflux disease (GERD)*, esophagitis results from acidic digestive juices flowing from the stomach backwards to the esophagus. In addition to symptoms of heartburn, the person who suffers with GERD may also experience excessive burping and frequent bouts of hiccups.

Over time, irritation and inflammation of the esophageal mucosa by stomach acid may lead to obstruction, narrowing, or cancer. Any of these conditions increases the risk of swallowing problems (especially aspiration, if food or liquid backs up into the throat).

Trauma or malignant disease within the chest (especially cancers of the esophagus or thyroid) can create an abnormal passageway between the trachea and the esophagus—a *tracheoesophageal fistula*. This can cause respiratory distress and pneumonia.

Swallowing and Fainting. Some persons with vagal hypersensitivity will experience so-called "swallow syncope." Food passing through the esophagus triggers a fainting episode (*syncope*) or lightheadedness. Swallow syncope can result from esophageal, cardiac, or other causes.

Effects of Aging

As noted earlier, our swallowing slows down as we grow older. Food, liquid, and pills take a little longer to travel from the mouth to the esophagus.

Chewing may become less effective with loss of muscle strength and limitation of jaw movement. The onset of airway protection and opening of the upper esophageal sphincter are delayed. In addition, there is a decrease in esophageal motility.

These changes are not generally a problem. Healthy older persons have not been found to aspirate more often than younger individuals. Such age-related changes, however, combined with the stresses of (1) a medical or neurologic disorder, (2) effects of medications used in their treatment, or (3) a lack of attention to safe swallowing will increase a person's risk of choking or aspiration.

Overview of
Causes of Swallowing Difficulty

Preparatory   Loss of smell or taste sensation; lack of saliva; weak chewing muscles; mouth pain; poorly-fitting dentures; lack of tongue control; mouth-breathing

Oral   Part of tongue missing; impaired tongue control; sensory loss

Pharyngeal   Absent or delayed reflex; muscle paralysis or weakness; sensory loss; diverticula; lack of coordination with breathing

Esophageal   Malfunction of upper or lower sphincters (achalasia, GERD); lack of esophageal motility; fistula; obstruction from inside or out

A Structural, Neurologic, Medical, or Psychologic Condition Can Act Any Phase

Now that we've looked at swallowing problems phase by phase, let's turn our attention to one of the most feared problems associated with swallowing: *choking*.

CHAPTER 4

WHAT TO DO
ABOUT CHOKING

WHAT TO DO
ABOUT CHOKING

The best thing to do about choking, of course, is to keep it from happening. That's a large part of what we're trying to do in this book.

Choking is scary. But it's not just anxiety-provoking. It accounts for thousands of deaths per year—with the elderly at highest risk.

By understanding the basics of swallowing and what can go wrong, you can take steps to reduce the risk of choking.

Unfortunately, it is not always going to be possible to prevent choking. So if you're assisting an elderly loved one at home, dining with friends at a restaurant, or eating by yourself, we want you to be able to recognize a choking emergency and deal with it effectively.

What Is Choking?

In everyday use, *choking*, *gagging*, and *coughing* while eating are often used interchangeably. In this book, we use the word *choking* specifically to refer to *airway obstruction*. That means (1) blockage of airflow to a person's lungs or (2) the person's signs of distress in response to such obstruction.

Since our lives depend upon a steady supply of oxygen, a blockage of any kind is important. Complete lack of oxygen causes brain damage after about four minutes and death within around ten.

Food, liquid, medication, or another object (e.g., a bottle cap) can block the *throat* to prevent air from getting *to* the airway (see Fig. 4-1). By contrast, an item lodged in the *esophagus* does not interfere with the supply of oxygen.

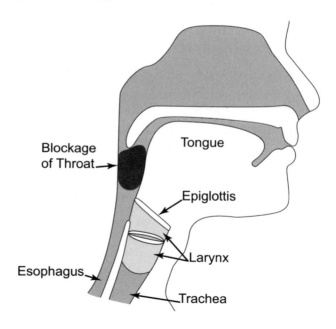

Figure 4-1: Blocking the Throat. An object blocks the throat, preventing air from getting *to* the airway.

Or an object gets into the trachea (the windpipe) itself, preventing air from getting *through* the airway (see Fig. 4-2).

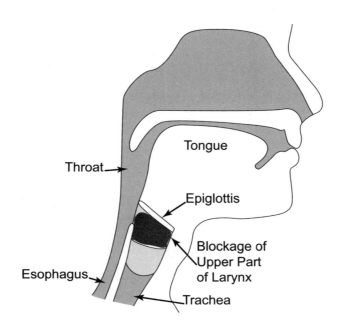

Figure 4-2: Blocking the Trachea. An object has entered the larynx ("voice box"), the uppermost part of the trachea, preventing breathing and talking.

It doesn't take much to block the airway. At its widest part, the larynx is slightly less than two inches in an adult male. The trachea below narrows to around one inch in diameter. So you can see how easily a meatball, a marshmallow, a bite of pickle, or even a large pill can obstruct the airway.

Risk Factors For Choking

The elderly are at highest risk of death by choking, even more so than young children. Several factors make them especially vulnerable.

Why the Elderly are at Increased Risk

- Missing teeth or having ill-fitting dentures
- Having several medical illnesses
- Having a neurologic disorder
- Taking medications with side effects that interfere with swallowing

---

Some people do not chew their food well enough. Autopsy results have yielded startlingly large pieces of unchewed steak the size of a deck of cards that block the airway.

Congestive heart failure and respiratory illnesses, among other medical conditions, can weaken a person and interfere with a vigorous, *protective* cough. Side effects of medication can also cause or contribute to swallowing difficulties (see Chapter 6).

With Parkinson disease, the whole swallowing process slows down. Coordination between breathing and swallowing is thrown off. Coughing is weak. See Chapter 3 for ways neurologic disorders at any age predispose to choking.

Choking Can Mimic a Heart Attack

A person choking on food can look like he's having a heart attack—especially if he is middle-aged or older. Unless it is recognized for what it is—a life-threatening choking incident—this "café coronary" can end a life as surely as a bona fide heart attack.

"Coronary" is short for *coronary occlusion* or *thrombosis*, a blockage of blood vessels that bring oxygen to the heart. This can cause a *heart attack*, or *myocardial infarction*.

When you suspect a heart attack, calling for emergency medical help (calling 911) is the right thing to do. But if a person is choking, you may need to carry out the Heimlich maneuver without delay.

The café coronary is, of course, not restricted to restaurants. It can happen in your own home or at your mother's. So be prepared.

"Café Coronary" vs. Heart Attack
(In a Conscious Person)

Choking episode .... Unable to speak or
  "café coronary"   breathe

Myocardial infarction ... Able to speak and
                              breathe

A Signal For Action

The choking person may have a *completely* or *partially* blocked airway. Either may require emergency intervention.

When the airway is completely blocked, a person will not be able to breathe, talk, or cough. His face will become gray or blue. His eyes may "bug out" in panic. He may collapse and lose consciousness.

When the airway is partially blocked, a person may be able to breathe—but only with difficulty or perhaps with a wheeze. If he can speak at all, his voice may be high-pitched, strained, noisy, or weak.

Blockage of Esophagus vs. Airway

When food feels "stuck"—like "it won't go down"—it can cause distress. This can be differentiated from choking because the person is able to speak and breathe. Ask the person: "Can you speak?"

Sometimes what is in the esophagus is vomited back up to the throat. From there it can be inhaled to obstruct the airway and create a choking emergency or be aspirated into the lungs.

Approach to the Choking Person

The choking person may give a sign of distress—a hand at their throat (see Fig. 4-3). When the person is unable to speak or breathe effectively, this calls for action.

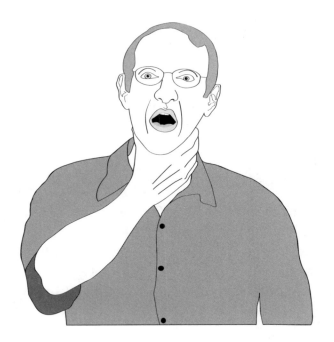

Figure 4-3: Choking Distress Signal. May be accompanied by turning blue, bulging eyes, running away in distress.

Ask the person, "Are you choking?" If he nods his head "Yes" or does not respond, act immediately. *Perform the Heimlich maneuver.*

Do *not* slap him on the back with the hope of dislodging the obstructing material. That could lodge the object more firmly against the airway or deeper in the trachea.

Do *not* reach into the throat to try and remove the obstructing food or other item. That wastes time and could push it in further.

If the person is able to cough, let him. That can by itself remove the obstruction. Hold off on your Heimlich maneuver for the time being.

Watch carefully. If the person is barely able to talk or breathe, get ready to administer the Heimlich maneuver. If you have an emergency alert device, activate it. Call 911 if necessary (for example, if the person collapses).

If a choking person—out of embarrassment or panic —leaves the dining area (whether at home or a restaurant) seeking privacy, *you must follow him!* Stay with him until the matter is resolved. A failure to see the incident through could be fatal (See Fig. 4-4).

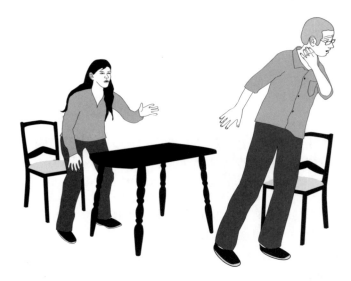

Figure 4-4: Follow That Person! The choking victim may leave the area to avoid embarrassment or out of panic. Follow and provide emergency treatment as needed.

The Heimlich Maneuver ("Abdominal Thrusts")

To perform the Heimlich maneuver on a conscious adult, get behind the choking person who is seated or standing. If seated, you will likely need to bend over or get on your knees. Otherwise, remain standing.

Wrap your arms around her waist. Place the thumb side of one fist against the upper abdomen above the umbilicus ("belly button") just below the sternum (the "breastbone"). Wrap your other hand around the pinky side of your fist (see Fig. 4-5).

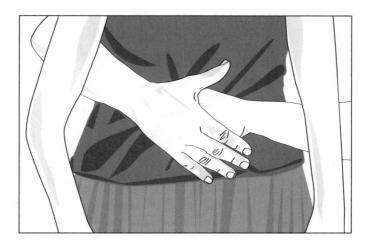

Figure 4-5: Hand Position For Heimlich Maneuver. Place the thumb side of your fist against the choking person's abdomen, between belly button and sternum. Then wrap the fist with your other hand.

With a quick, upward thrust, pull your hands toward yourself against the person's abdomen. You may actually lift the person off the chair or the floor. Repeat several times if necessary (see Fig. 4-6)

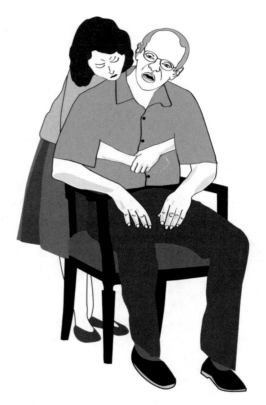

Figure 4-6: The Heimlich Maneuver. Carrying out the maneuver when the choking person is seated.

If the choking person collapses or is too large for you to get your arms around (for example, if a smaller person is rescuing a large adult), quickly lay the person down face up.

Open the person's mouth (with your thumb on his tongue, index finger under the chin). If you see an object and it is loose, remove it. Do not try to grasp an object lodged in the person's throat. This may push it further into the airway.

Get on your knees at the level of the upper thigh or hips and place the heel of your hand just above the umbilicus, below the rib cage. Place your free hand on the other. Press into the abdomen with quick, forward thrusts. Repeat several times as needed (see Fig. 4-7). If the airway clears and the person is still unresponsive, begin CPR.

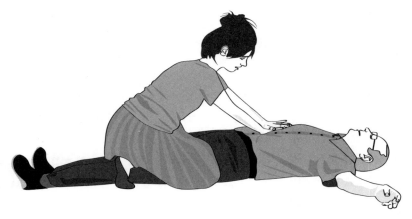

Figure 4-7: Victim on Floor. If the victim has collapsed or is too large, perform the Heimlich maneuver on the floor. Call 911 as soon as possible.

If another person is present, have her remove any food material that has been expelled into the mouth so it doesn't cause further blockage. If the person vomits, turn the entire body to one side to prevent aspiration. Remove the vomited material as quickly as possible.

If two or three attempts do not expel the obstructing object and restore breathing, continue the procedure and have someone call 911.

Alternatives to the Heimlich Maneuver

Some sources recommend sharp blows to the back or chest thrusts if abdominal thrusts do not work or even before the Heimlich maneuver. We follow the recommendations of the American Heart Association (AHA) as to clearing a blocked airway in a conscious adult or child one year of age or older, namely, proceeding directly to the Heimlich maneuver (abdominal thrusts).

The AHA (2010) states that "Although chest thrusts, back slaps, and abdominal thrusts are feasible and effective for relieving severe foreign-body airway obstruction in conscious (responsive) adults and children ≥1 year of age, for simplicity in training it is recommended that abdominal thrusts be applied in rapid sequence until the obstruction is relieved. If abdominal thrusts are not effective, the rescuer may consider chest thrusts..."

The Guidelines continue: "Chest thrusts should be used for obese patients if the rescuer is unable to encircle the victim's abdomen. If the choking victim is in the late stages of pregnancy, the rescuer should use chest thrusts instead of abdominal thrusts."

To learn and practice the most up-to-date techniques for CPR (cardiopulmonary resuscitation) in general and the approach to a choking person in particular, consult with your CPR specialist, the American Heart Association, or the American Red Cross.

Saving Your Own Life

You can choke while eating alone. For that reason, you need to know how to carry out the Heimlich maneuver on yourself.

If you choke and find yourself unable to speak, cough, or breathe, don't panic. If you have an emergency contact device, trigger it immediately. Carry out the Heimlich maneuver on yourself without delay.

Stand again a sink, countertop, desk, or sturdy chair. Press your upper belly firmly against its upper edge, grasping its sides with both hands. Thrust yourself forward vigorously, bending slightly at the waist. Repeat as needed (see Fig. 4-8).

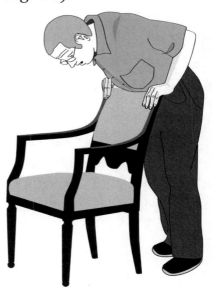

**Figure 4-8:
The Self-Heimlich
Maneuver.**
Use chair, desk,
countertop—or
your own fist.

If a desk or other suitable structure is not available, use your own wrapped fist to carry out the abdominal thrusts.

Why the Heimlich Maneuver Works

As Dr. Henry Heimlich explained some 40 years ago, choking is common when a person talks or laughs while swallowing food. The obstructing material prevents air from getting to—or through—the larynx ("voice box"), which is why a person cannot talk or breathe.

By pressing against the upper abdomen, between the umbilicus and the chest, you push the diaphragm upward into the chest, making the chest cavity smaller. This compresses the lungs, causing a strong flow of air out the airway—in essence, creating an artificial cough. The air flow carries the obstructing object out of the airway into, or out of, the mouth.

Post-Heimlich Check-Up

We recommend that after you have carried out the Heimlich maneuver on an ill or frail elderly person you take him or her straight away for medical examination to check for complications such as a broken rib or damage to an internal organ such as the liver or spleen.

Keep in mind that the object the person was choking on sometimes gets through to the lungs. Weeks, or even months, later the person may show symptoms of respiratory illness (such as pneumonia or lung abscess) arising from that incident.

What To Do About Choking

Prevention   Follow safe swallowing
strategies.
Be prepared for an emergency
at all times, especially
in persons with medical
or neurologic illness.
If concerned about choking,
seek swallowing evaluation.

Recognition Watch for choking distress
signal, inability to breathe
or talk, turning blue or
gray, agitation, leaving
the room in a panic.

Action   Follow the person.
Observe.
Let the person cough.
Perform the Heimlich
maneuver if necessary.
Activate emergency alert device.
Call 911.

Follow-Up Carry out post-Heimlich
medical checkup.
Watch for later
respiratory illness.

The next chapter deals with another complication of swallowing difficulty that can have a fatal outcome: *aspiration.*

CHAPTER 5

ASPIRATION AND PNEUMONIA

Aspiration And Pneumonia

Remember the time you were having lunch with a couple of friends. Chatting, laughing, having a pleasant afternoon. All of a sudden you had a violent coughing fit that brought tears to your eyes.

A minute or so later, when the attack subsided and everyone could breathe again, a friend asked: "What happened?"

"I think food went down the wrong tube," you said.

Definition of Aspiration

When food, medication, or liquid (including saliva) gets into the wrong tube—the airway instead of the esophagus—that's *aspiration* (see Fig. 5-1).

Because you were in good health, you got rid of the offending material by coughing vigorously. But what about your elderly aunt? She's not in the best of health—weak overall—and her cough is anything but strong.

If something gets into her airway, it has a good chance of getting to her lungs. That could be the ticket to pneumonia, deterioration, and death—a common sequence in frail, elderly persons and those with medical or neurologic illness such as congestive heart failure, COPD, Parkinson disease, multiple sclerosis, ALS, or stroke.

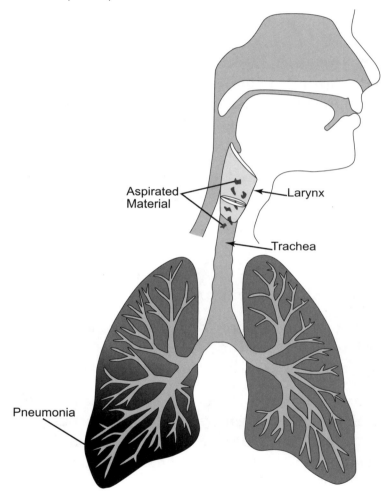

Figure 5-1: Aspiration and Pneumonia. Food, liquid (including saliva), or medication passes through the larynx to reach the lungs to cause pneumonia.

Aspiration vs. Penetration

To be more precise, *aspiration* is defined by material passing through the vocal cords, located within the larynx—the highly-specialized, uppermost part of the airway. Until that point, it's considered *penetration*.

That's probably what happened to you at lunch the other day unless you developed symptoms of respiratory illness. That would suggest *aspiration*. The material passed beyond your vocal cords to reach your lungs to cause pneumonia.

What Causes Aspiration

Aspiration can result from problems at any phase of the swallowing process:

- Lack of saliva or weak chewing muscles— anything that prevents formation of a proper bolus (*Preparatory*)
- A tongue under poor control, unable to transport the bolus effectively from mouth to throat (*Oral*)
- Lack of coordination between breathing and swallowing; a faulty swallowing reflex with incomplete palatal closure or weak pharyngeal muscles that can't push the food down (*Pharyngeal*)
- A scarred upper esophageal sphincter that doesn't open fully to permit the complete bolus to pass or a malfunctioning lower esophageal sphincter that stays closed so foodstuff can back up to the throat (*Esophageal*).

Symptoms of Unsafe Swallowing

These signs and symptoms during eating, drinking, or taking medication (especially when they occur repeatedly) suggest an unsafe swallow with increased risk of aspiration and pneumonia.

- coughing
- sputtering
- tearing of eyes
- runny nose (due to increased tearing)
- wheezing
- change in voice after the swallow (weak, hoarse, or gargly)
- need to swallow more than once
- tired out by eating
- feeling food is stuck in throat
- multiple bouts of pneumonia

Be aware that aspiration can take place *without any warning signs whatsoever*. That is called *silent aspiration*. We'll talk more about that later in this chapter.

Aspiration can happen any age. Especially vulnerable are those with neurologic or medical illnesses such as Parkinson disease, stroke, Alzheimer disease, Guillain-Barré syndrome, multiple sclerosis, head trauma, ALS, congestive heart failure, or COPD.

Aspiration and Pneumonia

Pneumonia caused by aspiration is called *aspiration pneumonia*. When saliva loaded with bacteria from the mouth, nose, or throat is aspirated into the lungs, it can cause bacterial pneumonia. Repeated episodes of aspiration associated with poor oral care increase the likelihood of bacterial pneumonia. (See *Oral Care Counts* in Chapter 8.)

Material aspirated from the stomach or esophagus usually has fewer bacteria but may contain irritating stomach acid. This stomach acid when aspirated can cause a chemical pneumonia, called *pneumonitis*.

Pneumonia vs. Pneumonitis

Pneumonitis and pneumonia typically arise in different kinds of clinical situations. *Aspiration pneumonitis* characteristically occurs in persons who have had a sudden and profound change in mental state.

For example, they may have experienced a generalized seizure, head injury, general anesthesia, drug overdose (including alcohol), or coma of any cause. Aspiration pneumonitis can also occur during the post-operative period, especially if the person is ill or frail.

Pneumonitis results from aspiration of acidic stomach contents. Thus it can occur with any medical, neurologic, or psychiatric illness associated with vomiting.

Aspiration pneumonia results from food, liquid (including saliva), or medication entering the airway and getting to the lungs to cause pneumonia.

The terms *pneumonia* and *pneumonitis* are often used interchangeably. Don't let the terminology confuse you. The take-home point in either case is that aspiration can cause a serious lung problem.

Typical symptoms of aspiration pneumonia include rapid, effortful breathing, cough, chest pain, wheezing, and fever. Elderly persons, however, may not have these typical symptoms of respiratory illness. Their pneumonia may declare itself by confusion, delirium, weakness, falling, or subnormal temperature.

The Cough as Clue

We tend to think of a cough as little more than an annoyance. A scratchy throat. Allergy. The beginning of a cold. Nothing to worry about.

By now, however, you know that cough may be the sign of a swallowing problem. We are *not* saying that every cough is due to aspiration. What we *are* saying, however, is that chronic cough (especially when it occurs during meals or while swallowing saliva), unexplained pneumonia, or signs and symptoms listed earlier in this chapter should alert you to the possibility of a swallowing problem.

An Unsettling Fact—Silent Aspiration

Aspiration does not always cause obvious symptoms. It can be silent—without coughing, throat-clearing, tearing, wheezing, voice change, or other symptoms.

Silent aspiration can occur while a person is awake or asleep. It can even occur in persons who receive tube feedings or are on a ventilator when saliva or regurgitated material is aspirated.

A Diagnostic Challenge

Even experienced swallowing specialists cannot definitively diagnose aspiration by observing a person at the bedside or in the office. They must combine the patient's history and clinical examination with specialized tests of swallowing (such as the modified barium swallow or fiberoptic endoscopy) that allow for direct visualization of the swallow (see Chapter 7).

That's why it is important for caregivers to keep the possibility of aspiration in mind when a loved one has a cough that won't go away or has been diagnosed with pneumonia more than once. Be aware that persons with Parkinson disease or acute stroke are at especially high risk of silent aspiration.

If you suspect silent aspiration, bring it up with your doctor or swallowing specialist.

Is Your Swallowing Unsafe?

Getting back to that unpleasant experience at lunch. Something like this can happen to anyone. If it has happened to you or a loved one even once, take note.

If you've experienced voice change, wheezing, pneumonia, or other symptoms of respiratory illness after

Overview of Aspiration

Definition	Food, drink, saliva, medication or stomach contents getting into the airway
Major Complications	Pneumonia; pneumonitis
Symptoms	Coughing, tearing, voice change, wheezing, fever, confusion, falling, none of the above
Diagnosis	In the office, at the bedside, by special investigation
Prevention and Early Detection	In elderly persons, any adult with a medical or neurologic disorder, yourself

a swallowing incident, consider aspiration a possible, if not likely, cause.

Is there something unsafe about *your* swallowing? What caused that nasty fit of coughing? Do you eat too quickly? Do you chew your food thoroughly? Do you have too much on your mind? Were you drinking alcohol? Were you laughing or talking and trying to swallow at the same time? Do you have an unrecognized medical or neurologic disorder?

Look at your eating habits. Make some changes if you need to. Consult with your doctor. That could save *your* life.

In the next chapter, we explore ways that medications—which are supposed to make things better—can make them *worse*.

CHAPTER 6

MEDICATION: A DOUBLE-EDGED SWORD

MEDICATION:
A DOUBLE-EDGED SWORD

A t times it seems as if the ill elderly are swimming in a sea of pills!

Let's look at your father. He has four major health problems: diabetes, Parkinson disease, COPD, and depression. His doctors have him on more than a dozen pills a day. That calls for a lot of organization—*and* a lot of swallowing.

Having a swallowing problem makes things even more complicated. Some of that medication could

How Medications Can Cause Swallowing Problems

- Reduce the supply of saliva
- Interfere with smell, taste, or appetite
- Cause drowsiness or inattention
- Irritate the throat or esophagus
- Allow overgrowth of harmful germs
- Cause swallowing muscles to tighten or weaken
- Slow passage of food through the esophagus
- Interfere with function of the lower esophageal sphincter

wind up burning his esophagus, getting sucked into his lungs, or interfering with his appetite to cause unwanted weight loss and weakness, increasing his risk of falling and, by suppressing his immune system, increasing his risk of infection.

More Pills, More Danger

The sheer number of pills can itself be a challenge. It requires a workable system to ensure that a person doesn't miss taking one medication and double up on another.

The challenge can be physical, too. Taking what feels like an endless round of pills can be time-consuming, fatiguing, anxiety-provoking, and just plain annoying. The first swallows may be fine—the last ones difficult and dangerous.

When a person takes multiple medications, the potential for side effects is magnified. Drugs are

Multiple Medications: Increased Risks

- Greater likelihood of medication error by patient, doctor, or pharmacist
- More opportunity to choke or aspirate
- Increased drug strength due to competition for breakdown
- Prolonged duration of action
- Fluid overload

metabolized by the liver and kidneys. When medications compete for breakdown and excretion, this can result in elevated blood levels and a longer stay in the body. Either of these can increase the risk of harmful side effects.

What Does "Anticholinergic" Mean?

When you read about side effects of medication, you will soon come across the word *anticholinergic*. It means "acting against *choline*," a shortened form of *acetylcholine*.

Acetylcholine ("uh-SEE-t'l-KOH-leen") is a chemical messenger, a neurotransmitter. Starting out in the brain, it is distributed widely throughout the body.

Anticholinergic Side Effects

Dry mouth	Eye pain
Sticky lips	Sensitivity to light
White-coated tongue	Urinary retention
Dehydration	Constipation
Loss of taste	Rapid heart rate
Decreased appetite	Dizziness
Fever	Memory loss
Red, hot skin	Confusion
Enlarged pupils	Agitation
Blurred vision	

In the brain, acetylcholine is involved in memory, in the mouth for salivation, in the skin for sweating, in the bladder for urination, in the eyes for vision, and in the gastrointestinal tract for moving food along. An anticholinergic drug thus can have a variety of effects.

Dry mouth (*xerostomia*) can be a troublesome anticholinergic side effect. It can make it difficult for pills to pass easily through the mouth, throat, or esophagus. Gelatinous capsules in particular can readily stick to their lining (*mucosa*) to cause a chemical burn or set up aspiration when the pill becomes unstuck.

Anticholinergic effects are not always negative. Sometimes they're desirable, as in the treatment of urinary incontinence, Parkinson disease, drooling, and irritable bowel syndrome. Belladonna preparations, for example, contain the potent anticholinergic agent *atropine*. This has long been used for treating intestinal cramps and diarrhea.

Belladonna: "Beautiful Lady"

In sixteenth century Italy, women applied a belladonna solution to their eyes to enlarge their pupils. It was felt to make them more attractive, hence, the name *bella donna*, Italian for *beautiful lady*.

Your mother at any age is beautiful. But if her pupils are unusually large, if she complains that light bothers her, if she has blurry vision, if she acts confused, or has memory loss, she may be suffering from the effects of one or more anticholinergic drugs.

"Natural" does not always mean "safe." Belladonna is derived from a plant known ominously as the *deadly nightshade*. Belladonna preparations—any anticholinergic medication for that matter—can be dangerous.

Acute toxicity can make a person "dry as a bone, blind as a bat, red as a beet, and mad as a hatter." These symptoms result from belladonna's ability to

- block saliva production,
- interfere with sweating,
- paralyze eye muscles involved in near vision,
- increase blood flow to the skin, and
- create mental disturbance.

It's easy to attribute confusion, memory loss, or other decline in an older person's mental state to "old age" or dementia. The culprit may, in fact, be anticholinergic (or other) medication.

Anticholinergics May Be Combined

Keep in mind that an anticholinergic drug may be used by itself or in combination with others (in a single pill). For example, the anticholinergic drug *orphenadrine* is sold as Norflex. Combined with aspirin and caffeine it becomes Norgesic.

Some Drugs With Anticholinergic Effects

Antivert	*meclizine*
Artane	*trihexyphenidyl*
Atarax	*hydroxyzine*
Atrovent	*ipratropium*
Benadryl	*diphenhydramine*
Bentyl	*dicyclomine*
Chlor-Trimeton	*chlorpheniramine*
Cogentin	*benztropine*
Compazine	*prochlorperazine*
Compoz	*diphenhydramine*
Ditropan	*oxybutynin*
Donnatal	*belladonna+phenobarbital*
Dramamine	*dimenhydrinate*
Elavil	*amitriptyline*
Flexeril	*cyclobenzaprine*
Haldol	*haloperidol*
Levsin	*hyoscyamine*
Norflex	*orphenadrine*
Nytol	*diphenhydramine*
Periactin	*cyproheptadine*
Phenergan	*promethazine*
Polaramine	*chlorpheniramine*
Pro-Banthine	*propantheline*
Quinidex	*quinidine*
Robinul	*glycopyrrolate*
Sinequan	*doxepin*
Spiriva	*tiotropium*
Thorazine	*chlorpromazine*
Vistaril	*hydroxyzine*

Some people may be taking more than one anticholinergic drug at the same time. They might, for example take *diphenhydramine* (Benadryl) for allergies and *amitriptyline* (Elavil) for pain or depression—thus compounding the likelihood of side effects.

Be on the alert. Anticholinergic drugs are everywhere. A partial list is included here. See Appendix C for a listing of anticholinergic drugs by therapeutic category.

Additional Drugs Causing Dry Mouth

Be aware that drugs that are not in the anticholinergic family can also cause dry mouth (*xerostomia*). These include *amphetamines* (Adderall, Dexedrine), cancer chemotherapeutic drugs, *carbamazepine* (Tegretol), *gabapentin* (Neurontin), *hydromorphone* (Dilaudid), *meperidine* (Demerol), *methylphenidate* (Ritalin, Concerta, Metadate, Quillivant), *oxycodone* (Oxycontin), and *topiramate* (Topamax).

By interfering with production of saliva and causing dry mouth, these and other drugs not only interfere with bolus formation and smooth passage through the mouth, throat, and esophagus, but they may also cut down on (1) immunoglobulins that help defend against disease and (2) enzymes that start the process of digestion in the mouth.

Other Drugs, Other Effects

Sense of Smell. A wide variety of medications are reported to reduce the sense of smell, which itself can reduce the supply of saliva. These include *cholestyramine* (Questar), *cimetidine* (Tagamet), *gentamicin* (Gentacin), *levodopa* (Sinemet), *nifedipine* (Procardia), *phenylephrine* (Neo-Synephrine), *promethazine* (Phenergan), and *propylthiouracil* (PTU).

Taste Sensation. Drugs reported to interfere with the sense of taste include *alprazolam* (Xanax), *amitriptyline* (Elavil), *ampicillin*, *azathioprine* (Imuran), *baclofen* (Lioresal), *carbamazepine* (Tegretol), *colchicine*, *diltiazem* (Cardizem), *doxepin* (Sinequan), *ethacrynic acid* (Edecrin), *hydrochlorothiazide* (Hydrodiuril), *hyoscyamine* (Levsin), *insulin*, *levodopa/carbidopa* (Sinemet, Parcopa), *lithium* (Lithobid), *methotrexate*, *nitroglycerin*, *prednisone*, *propranolol* (Inderal), *spironolactone* (Aldactone), *sulfasalazine* (Azulfidine), and *vincristine*.

Level of Alertness. Drugs for agitation, allergies, anxiety, sleep, pain, and psychosis may cause drowsiness or interfere with crucial coordination between breathing and swallowing. Included in this group are *lorazepam* (Ativan), *olanzapine* (Zyprexa), *diphenhydramine* (Benadryl), *diazepam* (Valium), *zolpidem* (Ambien), *oxycodone* (OxyContin), *hydrocodone* (Vicodin), and *thioridazine* (Mellaril).

Muscle Movement. Several phenothiazines (antipsychotic drugs)—including *chlorpromazine* (Thorazine) and *thioridazine* (Mellaril)—have been associated with swallowing problems, specifically choking. This has been linked with their effects upon muscle. They can, for example, cause too little movement (a Parkinson-like syndrome) or too much movement (tardive dyskinesia).

Microenvironment. Antibiotics used to treat infectious diseases (such as pneumonia or urinary tract infection) and drugs for cancer can alter the balance of microorganisms that normally live in the gastrointestinal tract, including the mouth. This can allow overgrowth of germs such as *Candida*, resulting in a painful yeast infection of the mouth called *thrush*.

Drug-Nutrient Interactions. Medications can cause problems in several ways. These include (1) blocking absorption, (2) enhancing elimination, and (3) interfering with the chemical activity of a nutrient once it has been absorbed. Resulting malnutrition and weakness can cause or worsen a swallowing problem.

Interference with absorption can reduce levels of vitamins (such as folic acid and other B vitamins, A, C, D, K, and carotene) and minerals (including iron, zinc, calcium, sodium, phosphate, and potassium). Drugs that may have these effects include *aluminum hydroxide* (Amphojel), *aspirin, cholestyramine* (Questran), *colchicine* (Colcrys), *lansoprazole* (Prevacid), *mineral oil*, and *omeprazole* (Prilosec).

Be Kind To Your Esophagus

The esophagus is especially vulnerable to medication effects. Certain drugs can

- slow the movement of food, liquid, or medication through the esophagus
- irritate its lining to cause ulceration and scarring and
- keep the lower esophageal sphincter from closing, allowing acidic stomach contents to flow back to the esophagus.

A pill that remains in the esophagus longer than the usual eight to twenty seconds can injure its lining (*mucosa*). Complications of such irritative, pill-induced esophagitis include bleeding, ulceration, and even perforation.

Damage to the esophageal mucosa can build up over months to years to cause a *stricture*, an encircling scar that interferes with passage of a bolus. Eating certain foods when one has such a stricture can cause pain that leads to a fainting spell (*syncope*).

Chest discomfort or shoulder pain can signal esophageal injury. Keep in mind that these can be symptoms of a heart attack as well. Don't put off contacting your doctor or emergency medical services if the situation calls for it.

Some medications cause the lower esophageal sphincter (LES) to relax at the wrong time. Recall that the LES is usually closed. This prevents acidic stomach contents from flowing back into the esoph-

Drugs Known To Cause Esophageal Damage

alendronate	Fosamax
aspirin	ASA, acetylsalicylic acid
doxycycline	Vibramycin
erythromycin	Ery Tab
ibuprofen	Advil, Motrin
indomethacin	Indocin
iron	Feosol, Slow Fe
naproxen sodium	Aleve, Naprosyn
potassium chloride	Kay Ciel, Slow-K
prednisone	Sterapred
quinidine	Quinidex
risedronate	Actonel
tetracycline	Panmycin, Sumycin
theophylline	Theo-Dur
vitamin C	ascorbic acid

agus (where it can damage the mucosa) and getting to the throat (from which it can be aspirated to cause pneumonitis).

Medications that promote relaxation of the lower esophageal sphincter include *anticholinergic drugs* (such as Elavil), *benzodiazepines* (including Valium), *aminophylline, nitroglycerin,* and beta-adrenergic agents such as *albuterol* (Proventil, Ventolin), *ipratropium* (Atrovent), and *terbutaline* (Brethine).

A Therapeutic Tightrope

The doctor often walks a fine line between therapeutic effects—such as relief of gastrointestinal distress, bronchial spasm, or muscular rigidity—and annoying or potentially dangerous side effects.

- Dry mouth can pave the way for a life-ending choking incident.
- Blurry vision can lead to a trip and fatal fall.
- Rapid pulse can cause cardiac decompensation and a heart attack.

Ask your pharmacist—or check online yourself—for side effects and interactions of prescribed and over-the-counter medications as well as herbal remedies. Write down your questions and concerns and discuss these with your doctor. (See **RESOURCES: Drug Information.**)

Making Pill-Taking Easier and Safer

The form of a medication may itself be a problem.

- Large pills (little "boulders") can get stuck traveling through the pharynx and esophagus.
- They may get into the trachea (to cause choking) or the lungs (to cause aspiration pneumonia).
- Gelatin capsules can stick to the throat, especially when the mouth is dry, and later be sucked into the lungs.
- Quick-dissolving medicines such as aspirin tablets without enteric coating can chemically burn the esophagus.

- Small pills can hide out in pockets between cheek and gum or where a tooth is missing, ready to be aspirated.

Ask your swallowing specialist or pharmacist if you can replace a problem medication with one that is better suited for your loved one. Keep in mind (1) the particulars of their swallowing problem and (2) their degree of understanding.

For example, it may be possible to replace a pill with liquid medication or one that dissolves in the mouth ("disintegrates") within a minute or less. Is the pill available in a smaller size or different shape? Can it

Special Care with Liquid Medication

If you're instructed to "Shake well before using," be sure to follow this advice. The active part of the medication can settle to the bottom of the bottle after a few hours on the shelf or in the medicine cabinet.

If you don't shake the bottle well, the first doses will be diluted while the last will be concentrated. You'll be undertreating at the top of the bottle, overdosing at the bottom. For example, with Dilantin, a seizure medication, this can mean seizures vs. wobbly walking.

So, for liquid medication, the mantra is "Shake It. Shake It, Baby!"

be crushed and sprinkled onto applesauce, pudding, or yogurt? (For persons with diabetes or high blood pressure, be sure to keep an eye on the sugar and salt content of commercially prepared applesauce and pudding.)

Don't chop first and ask later. Some medicines, such as a long-acting form of *carbamazepine* (Tegretol), are designed to work as a *whole pill only*. Cut it in half and you destroy the drug-delivery system.

Tips For Taking Medication

Here are some suggestions that can make pill-taking easier and safer.

- Be calm.
- Breathe in a relaxed manner.
- Make sure your mouth is moist.
- Take one pill at a time.
- Place the pill toward the front of your tongue to reduce the tendency to gag.
- Take a good sip of water.
- Hold the pill and liquid in your mouth for a second or two before swallowing.
- Tip chin to chest while swallowing.
- Swallow consciously and forcefully.
- Relax between swallows and give yourself credit for a job well done.

Some medications bypass the oral route entirely. They are given as a suppository, by skin patch, by inhalation, or by injection.

A technique known as *effortful swallow* can help in taking pills (or for swallowing in general). This technique makes swallowing more consciously forceful. You are asked to concentrate, use your voluntary muscles, and *"Swallow hard!"*—like you're trying to swallow a golf ball.

Pill-Taking Anxiety

Fear can make taking medication an ordeal. The trauma of a childhood choking incident may extend into adulthood to cause difficulty swallowing pills.

If your uncle expects to have a problem getting his pills down, it is likely he will. In the blink of an eye he's anxious and aroused, ready for fight-or-flight. His mouth is dry, his throat tight. None of this is conducive to swallowing safely.

Before concluding that a swallowing problem is psychological, the doctor needs to consider and rule out neurologic and structural causes of swallowing difficulty. *Myasthenia gravis*, for example, is notorious for being misdiagnosed as *hysteria* or other emotional disorder.

For swallowing problems found to be emotionally-based—as can occur in persons with post-traumatic stress disorder (PTSD)—the speech-language pathologist will (1) work with the patient (and caregivers) to increase knowledge and awareness of swallowing, (2) develop strategies that reduce the fear of swallowing, and (3) collaborate with a mental health professional.

One at a Time

Taking one pill at a time can be a nuisance, we know. But it's for your own safety.

Be aware, however, that this can add up to significant fluid intake over the course of a day. That's something to keep in mind when a person has kidney disease or a heart condition and needs to keep a close eye on their fluids.

Check with your doctor as to how much water you are allowed so you don't get fluid overloaded. A cup designed to deliver a pre-determined amount of fluid per sip (5 or 10 cc) may be of help in these situations.

It's *Not* Cool

It may look good on TV or in the movies, but you should not throw your head back and toss pills to the back of your throat. They might wind up in your airway—and you in the hospital.

(Under some circumstances, the swallowing specialist may recommend that the head be tilted back —but without a pill toss, of course.)

If you need to tip your head back to get water from a cup or bottle, make sure you return to a level position before swallowing so you don't increase your risk of aspirating.

If you take pride in swallowing pills without water, be aware that this, too, is like playing with fire. It's a great way to set yourself up for choking or esophageal damage.

Always take pills with water or other liquid. (Applesauce or yogurt may be a suitable alternative.) Saliva is not enough. Once again, don't dry swallow pills!

Earlier If Possible

Try to schedule medication for as early in the day as possible, not right before bedtime. Lying down immediately after taking medication will likely increase the risk of acid reflux and pills irritating the esophagus.

While you're awake, up and about, you swallow saliva more often than when you're asleep. That helps move things through the esophagus. So, after taking medication, sit or, if permitted, walk for a few minutes.

Taking Medication Safely

- Be aware of side effects and drug interactions.
- Take the right pill at the right time.
- Take one pill at a time with liquid or suitable alternative.

- Take medication in most suitable form: pills, liquid, crushed and sprinkled, orally disintegrating.
- Watch out for fluid overload.
- Watch for side effects (such as dry mouth or drowsiness).
- Don't toss or dry-swallow pills.
- Shake liquid medication vigorously before use.
- Give by non-oral route (skin patch, suppository, inhaler, injection) when indicated.
- Use the effortful swallow technique (if recommended).
- Watch for pills left behind after the swallow.
- For anxiety, work with a mental health professional and a swallowing specialist.
- Take medication earlier in the day when possible, not at bedtime.
- Don't lie down right after taking medication.
- Review medications regularly with your doctor.
- Discontinue medications no longer needed.

In the next chapter, we discuss how to get help if you suspect a swallowing problem.

CHAPTER 7

GETTING HELP

Getting Help

At this point, you probably have a sense as to whether your mother, your father, your spouse—or *you*—have a swallowing problem. If you haven't begun the process of evaluation and treatment, now is the time to take action. We will show you how.

In this chapter, we will guide you in gathering your concerns and observations so you can get the help you need. We've put together a *Letter For Your Doctor* you can use to record key information (Appendix A). How long have you been worried about swallowing? What has prompted your concern? Have you noticed frequent throat-clearing or coughing with meals, a voice change after eating, or the feeling that the food won't go down?

The *Letter For Your Doctor* allows you to list medical problems, hospitalizations, and medications. Fill out the *Letter* with your spouse, another family member, a friend, a professional caregiver, or by yourself. Keep a copy.

Bring the *Letter* to your next doctor's visit. Or, even better, get it to your primary medical provider (internist, geriatrician, family physician, general practitioner, nurse practitioner, or physician assistant) *now*, before the next scheduled visit.

This may prompt the doctor to see you sooner than previously scheduled. Or he may feel you should see a swallowing specialist right away.

Even if your appointment is for tomorrow, if things worsen—in terms of difficulty swallowing, labored breathing, or progressive weakness—contact your doctor immediately, go to your local emergency room, or call 911.

The Swallowing Specialist

The doctor may refer you to a *speech therapist,* or *speech-language pathologist.* "But," you say, "there's nothing wrong with my speech!"

True enough (perhaps). But it turns out that many of the structures we use for *speaking* (including the mouth, tongue, lips, and throat) are also used for *swallowing* (as well as for *breathing*). Thus, the assessment and treatment of swallowing problems falls within the realm of speech-language pathology.

The speech-language pathologist (SLP) will have the initials CCC-SLP after her or his name. They stand for Certificate of Clinical Competence in Speech-Language Pathology.

This certification means that she (or he) has successfully completed a rigorous graduate training program (two to three years for a master's degree, more for a

Ph.D.) followed by an additional year of supervised clinical fellowship. The SLP has also passed a national qualifying examination with certification through the American Speech-Language-Hearing Association (ASHA) and is licensed to practice in your state.

Speech-language pathologists work in a wide variety of settings. These include hospitals, nursing homes, rehab centers, patients' residences, or private offices. Some speech-language pathologists have made swallowing an area of special expertise, achieving BCS-S certification through the American Board of Swallowing and Swallowing Disorders.

History of the Swallowing Problem

Developing a treatment plan requires characterizing as specifically as possible your swallowing problem. The speech-language pathologist will begin with a detailed history of your swallowing.

It will include your state of medical health, medications, food habits, educational background, family structure, and support system. All are pertinent to the diagnosis and management of your swallowing problem.

Many of the symptoms associated with swallowing difficulty are listed in the *Letter For Your Doctor* (Appendix A). These include

- coughing or clearing the throat frequently while eating
- tearing of the eyes, runny nose, or voice change during meals

- the feeling that food won't go down
- pneumonia (especially if recurrent)
- excessive burping (belching)
- chronic hiccups
- weight loss or
- falls.

The SLP will also use your observations to clarify what kinds of liquids, solids, or pills you do well with or give you difficulty.

Your medical condition plays a key role in the diagnosis and treatment of your swallowing problem. With chronic illnesses such as COPD, esophageal disorders, Parkinson disease, ALS, or multiple sclerosis, a swallowing problem may occur at any time. This may already have led to dehydration, malnutrition, or aspiration pneumonia.

Persons with stroke, head trauma, upper cervical injury, or Guillain-Barré syndrome, for example, may develop swallowing problems acutely.

Sometimes a swallowing problem will be the first symptom of a previously undiagnosed disorder. This can occur, for example, with myasthenia gravis, ALS, multiple sclerosis, cancer, botulism, or diphtheria.

Swallowing problems may surface years after illness or trauma such as with post-polio syndrome and post-traumatic stress disorder (PTSD), for example, among war veterans or in persons who have been sexually abused.

Medications, as we have seen, can interfere with the swallowing process at any phase. Reduced alertness (with anti-anxiety medication), cutting down on saliva production (with anticholinergics), interfering with movement of pharyngeal muscles (with some antipsychotic drugs), and "burning" the esophagus (with osteoporosis pills) are but a few of the ways that drugs can have a negative impact on swallowing.

General Examination

These are some of the questions the SLP will address:

- Are you alert or drowsy?
- Oriented to person, place, time, and situation?
- Are you calm? Depressed? Anxious?
- Focused or easily distracted?
- How is your memory for recent and past events?
- Are you able to learn new information?
- How is your hearing for conversation?
- Are you breathing comfortably through your nose or effortfully through your mouth?
- Is your breathing shallow, rapid, or labored?
- Do you have a cough or wheeze?
- How is your posture? Are you hunched over at the shoulders or tilted to one side?
- Does one side of your face droop?
- How do your head, shoulders, neck, arms, and hands move?
- Do you appear underweight or overweight?

- Are your lips sticky, dry, or chapped?
- Are you drooling?
- Is your voice strong and full, or weak and nasal?
- Is your speech fluent and easy to understand?
- Do you have a vocal tremor?
- Do you understand the questions being asked?
- Do you have insight as to your current medical condition?
- Do you have difficulty swallowing your saliva? Does it pool in your throat?
- Do you think you have a swallowing problem?
- What foods, liquids, or medications give you trouble?
- Does it appear that you will need a caregiver to provide assistance once a treatment plan is developed?

The SLP may take your vital signs: pulse, blood pressure, respiratory rate, and temperature.

This will guide her in choosing the most suitable exercises. For example, some exercises may be unsafe for persons with high (or low) blood pressure, cardiac conditions, or respiratory problems.

Oral Motor Examination

The SLP will observe and record the following:

What is the overall state of your oral health? Are teeth missing? Are your dentures securely in place?

Is your tongue moist? Do you have "bad breath" (*halitosis*)? Are your cheeks a healthy pink on the inside or marked by white patches or other discoloration?

The *oral motor examination* focuses on the muscles involved in swallowing. These include muscles of the face, lips, tongue, jaw, soft palate, throat, and larynx.

After examining these structures, she will assess the strength, coordination, speed, range of motion, and accuracy of movement. Each one of these elements of motor function plays a role in swallowing. Hence, the oral motor examination will guide the specialist as to the cause (or causes) of your swallowing problem and a plan for treatment.

She may ask you to open your mouth, stick out your tongue, puff out your cheeks, make various facial gestures, and imitate sounds. She will check your gag reflex and the sensation of your face and within your mouth.

She will take note of your *breathing* and your *voice*. Is your breathing effortful? Rapid? Shallow? Are you wheezing? Do you get short of breath when you speak? Is your voice hoarse, weak, or nasal? Is your speech clear or garbled? Do you cough or clear your throat when talking?

Next comes evaluation of *cough*. The SLP will assess the strength and effectiveness of your cough and your ability to clear your throat. Both are important for airway protection.

A Trial Swallow

Next comes an examination of swallowing itself—if it is considered safe to do so: a *trial swallow*. You will be offered small amounts of food or liquid of different textures to observe how you handle them.

The purpose of the trial swallow is to

1. see if this brings out the swallowing problem,
2. guide treatment recommendations, and
3. suggest additional testing (as needed) to obtain more specific information about your swallowing problem.

The trial swallow can detect swallowing problems that occur during the *oral phase*. For swallowing problems that occur during the *pharyngeal* or *esophageal phases*, further testing is generally necessary.

Be aware that having a few sips of water at the doctor's office is not an adequate test for a swallowing problem. It may be erroneously interpreted and lead to inappropriate recommendations.

The therapist cannot rely upon a trial swallow to diagnose (or exclude) silent aspiration because—by definition—that occurs without symptoms or signs of swallowing difficulty such as coughing or throat-clearing.

The examination may include monitoring changes in oxygen level (*oxygen saturation*) during the swallow. This measurement is obtained simply and non-invasively by placing a sensor around your finger. Results are available immediately. A decrease in oxygen saturation during or after the swallow may suggest further evaluation.

What the Therapist Looks For

These are some of the things the SLP will look for:

- Did your swallow appear to be safe and effective?
- Did it hurt to swallow?
- Did you cough or clear your throat before, during, or after the swallow?
- Did your voice become weak, hoarse, or gurgly after the swallow?
- Did your eyes tear or your nose run afterwards?
- Were you aware of any of these difficulties?
- Did you feel that the food got stuck on the way down? If so, where?
- Did your Adam's apple rise fully and move forward with the swallow?
- Did you need more than one swallow to get the food or liquid down?
- Were you more comfortable with solids or liquids? What kinds of liquids—thin like water, or thicker as with tomato juice?

- Did food remain on your tongue, stuck to your cheeks, or in your throat after you swallowed?
- Were you aware of it? Did you sweep your mouth with your tongue?
- How well were you able to coordinate breathing and chewing? Breathing and swallowing?

A word or two about a "gurgly" or "gargly" voice. When food or liquid remains in the throat after an attempted swallow, air pushed up from the lungs through the larynx has to travel through this material. This can result in a bubbly, rattling sound. The material left behind can be aspirated into the lungs when breathing resumes after the swallow.

Immediate Treatment and Further Testing

The swallowing specialist may recommend that protective measures be put into place at once because of immediate dangers of choking or aspiration. These might include safe swallowing strategies such as therapeutic positioning, swallowing maneuvers, or a change in diet texture.

She might also recommend referral to a medical specialist (neurologist, pulmonologist, or ear-nose-and-throat specialist, for example).

Chest X-Ray

A chest x-ray is *not* a test of a swallowing problem. Your doctor may send you for a chest x-ray to look for pneumonia that may have resulted from aspiration.

A particular pattern on the x-ray can suggest aspiration as the cause of pneumonia. More than one bout of pneumonia with an aspiration pattern suggests a significant swallowing problem.

In conclusion, if the chest x-ray is normal, don't assume that all is well with swallowing and that aspiration has been ruled out. Once again, the chest x-ray is *not* a test of swallowing.

Modified Barium Swallow Study

In order to identify where your swallowing breaks down, especially when aspiration is of concern, your speech-language pathologist may refer you for a *modified barium swallow* study (*MBS*). Also known as *videofluoroscopy*, the MBS is the standard test for viewing the structure and function of the mouth, throat, and larynx during the swallow.

The MBS looks at the anatomy and physiology of the oral and pharyngeal stages of swallowing—how they appear and how they work. It can (1) confirm the clinical suspicion of aspiration, (2) clarify at what phase (or phases) the swallowing process breaks down, (3) determine what foods and liquids in what amounts you handle best, and (4) identify postures and maneuvers that facilitate safe swallowing.

More on the MBS

Barium is a chalky, white material that—mixed with food or liquid—allows the food or liquid being swallowed to show up on x-ray. A radiologist and a speech-language pathologist carry out the MBS study. During the test, you will be asked to swallow varying amounts of food and liquid—a cookie or applesauce, for example—mixed with barium.

If you aspirate or have difficulty swallowing during the test, the SLP may ask you to carry out maneuvers such as changes in head position during the swallow to see if these make your swallow safer and more effective.

The procedure is painless and non-invasive. It usually takes thirty minutes to an hour to complete. The entire swallowing process is recorded digitally or on videotape for review, interpretation, and treatment planning.

Other Tests of Swallowing

The *barium swallow* is the standard test for looking at the esophageal phase of swallowing. It does not assess the pharyngeal phase. Thus it is not a test that looks at airway protection—a crucial aspect of swallowing safely.

When there is a risk of aspiration, it is safer to have the *modified barium swallow* first, since the barium *swallow* requires the patient to swallow a relatively large amount of barium liquid, which itself can be aspirated.

Fiberoptic endoscopic examination of swallowing (*FEES*) is used to look primarily at the pharyngeal phase of swallowing. It does not involve x-rays. A specialist passes a small, thin endoscope—a tube containing a tiny camera—through the nose (which some people may not be able to tolerate).

This allows for direct visualization of the larynx and the pharyngeal phase of swallowing. A limitation of this test is a brief lack of clear image ("whiteout") as the swallowing reflex is triggered.

Esophageal endoscopy (which may be combined with biopsy) may be carried out to evaluate esophagitis or suspected esophageal cancer.

Your speech-language pathologist will recommend which test or tests to carry out depending upon the particulars of your swallowing problem and the pros and cons of each technique.

Practical Considerations Worldwide

We realize that under some circumstances it is not possible to have an instrumental examination (such as MBS or FEES) carried out in a timely manner, if at all.

As articulated by the World Gastroenterology Organisation, dysphagia is a common problem throughout the world. Diagnostic (and therapeutic) options will depend upon a country or region's resources. It classifies these options as ranging from "limited" to "state of the art."

Clinicians will establish a working diagnosis based upon the history and examination (which may include a trial swallow). From there they will develop a treatment program designed to lessen the risk of aspiration (as well as choking, malnutrition, and dehydration).

The Swallowing Team

In addition to your speech-language pathologist, other specialists often take part in the evaluation and treatment of persons with possible or identified swallowing problems. They might include one or more of the following: an ear-nose-and-throat (ENT) specialist, neurologist, oncologist, pulmonologist, gastroenterologist, rheumatologist, psychiatrist, or dentist.

The team may also include a physical therapist (to work on body posture, balance, strength, and breathing), an occupational therapist (to guide patients and caregivers in the mechanics of eating and other activities of daily living), a nurse, a nutritionist, and a pharmacist.

It is important that aides and caregivers, too, be involved, as they need to understand their role in carrying out the treatment plan.

Cultural Differences

When dealing with your swallowing specialist and other members of the team, it is crucial that the clinical process is carried out within the appropriate cultural context.

Communication is of paramount importance at all stages, especially when it comes to quality-of-life and end-of-life matters. Religious, personal, and spiritual beliefs must be an integral part of the treatment plan.

Overview of the Clinical Process

History of swallowing problem

Current and past medical, neurologic, and
     psychiatric history

Medication list

Bedside/office examination of swallowing

Investigation (as indicated) by MBS, FEES, or
     other test

Treatment (positioning, swallowing
     maneuvers, exercises, diet modification,
     prosthesis, surgery)

Referral (pulmonary, ENT, neurology, other)

Follow-up examination and re-evaluation

Modification of treatment plan as needed

The next chapter looks at the *treatment of swallowing problems.*

CHAPTER 8

TREATING SWALLOWING PROBLEMS

Treating Swallowing Problems

Treatment is not "one size fits all." Based upon a comprehensive swallowing evaluation, treatment is individually tailored to meet the needs of your loved one. The swallowing specialist will look at the particulars of the swallowing problem and come up with specific treatment options.

The goals of treatment are to

- get to a state where swallowing is accomplished as safely as possible (minimizing the risks of choking or aspiration),
- ensure adequate nutrition and hydration, and
- accomplish the first two goals as pleasantly as possible.

Treatment does not take place in a vacuum. It involves the whole person as well as the family or other support system. Anything that improves a person's overall condition—strength, stamina, motivation, and emotional state—is likely to help with swallowing. And a safe, reliable swallow is likely to help overall condition.

The treatment plan for a swallowing problem will take into account five bodily systems. These systems

—individually or in combination—may cause or contribute to dysphagia:

- neurologic
- muscular
- cardiorespiratory
- gastrointestinal
- cognitive/emotional.

The treatment plan begins with an *understanding* of what is wrong with the swallow and why. By this point, you should have a basic knowledge of swallowing, a sense of where things can go wrong, and for what reason(s):

- a medical condition (e.g., congestive heart failure or pulmonary disease)
- a neurologic disorder (e.g., stroke or Parkinson disease)
- a structural problem (e.g., part of the tongue missing due to cancer surgery)
- complicating effects of medication (e.g., dry mouth or altered sense of smell).

The Setting for Meals

Whatever the swallowing issues may be, the setting of the meal is important. Close doors to reduce traffic (grandchildren, pets, repairmen, or others).

If your loved one is easily distracted, turn off the TV and keep mealtime conversation to a minimum. It's perfectly fine to provide reminders to chew thoroughly or carry out a particular swallowing maneuver. Don't forget to silence your cell phone and catch up with email and text messages later.

We're not advocating a somber atmosphere. But be careful about cracking jokes during a meal. Laughter (even talking) alters a person's breathing pattern and can cause an unsafe swallow.

Obviously, a person shouldn't eat (or be fed) if sleepy, confused, or agitated. Likewise, don't try to feed someone who is unusually weak or out of breath.

Proper Positioning During and After Meals

Sitting upright, not tilted back or slumped to the side, helps breathing and swallowing. Sitting stably, feet on the floor if possible, also facilitates eating.

If your mother takes her meals in bed, have her sit as upright as possible. Make sure her head does not fall back. Place pillows at her sides and behind her head so her trunk and head are straight.

Positioning after the meal is important, too. Don't rush your father to bed. A person should remain upright or nearly so for thirty to forty-five minutes after eating or taking medication. This puts gravity to work, helping move the bolus through the esophagus and into the stomach. In that way you reduce the likelihood that refluxed material will be aspirated.

Even if your loved one takes medication for reflux, don't count on that being one hundred percent effective. At bedtime, elevate the upper part of the body

30 degrees by placing wedge pillows at the top of the bed to reduce the risk of reflux and aspiration during sleep.

Being Careful with Problem Foods

Avoid foods that have caused problems in the past. These may include steak, crusty bread or toast, popcorn, raw vegetables, whole nuts, bananas, peanut butter, horseradish, highly spiced foods, pickles, or pastries dusted with sugar.

Watch out for foods of *mixed consistency*. A mouthful of food may contain both liquid and solid textures. That can make swallowing tricky.

Consider dry cereal with milk. Your uncle may be able to handle dry, crunchy cornflakes alone without a problem. But when combined with milk, the liquid flows willy-nilly to the back of his throat, causing him to cough and aspirate (see Fig. 8-1).

The solution may simply be to give the cornflakes time to get soft. Less crunch, greater safety.

What about salad? It certainly looks harmless. But salad can be hazardous for several reasons. It can be difficult to reduce lettuce to a pasty, manageable bolus. Pieces stick to the tongue, hide out in the throat, or get trapped between cheek and gum in a position to be aspirated.

Salad dressing is an additional concern. As with milk and dry cereal, the vinaigrette can rush ahead of the lettuce to an unprotected airway and be sucked into the lungs with the next breath.

Likewise, be careful with fruit. It, too, is often of mixed texture. Take a grape, for example. It is made up of skin, pulp, pit, and juice. All four must be reckoned with when it comes to chewing and swallowing safely.

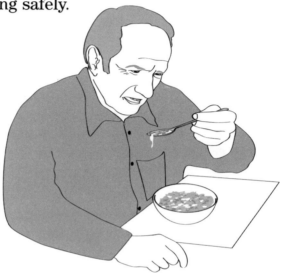

Figure 8-1: A Breakfast Challenge. Foods of mixed consistency—such as dry cereal with milk—can be dangerous.

Keep in mind that ice cream and some gelatin preparations start out in a relatively solid state. But in a serving dish, in a spoon, or in the mouth, they melt to become a thin liquid—which may be difficult for your loved one to handle.

Watch out, too, for carbonated beverages, which combine water and gas. Bubbles can tickle the throat to cause coughing or sneezing that interferes with the coordination of breathing and swallowing. (On the other hand, carbonated beverages may be included in the treatment plan because of the sensory stimulation they provide to the mouth and throat.)

This list is not exhaustive. These are a few examples that illustrate the complexity and importance of taking into account various food textures and making adjustments that will lessen the risk of aspiration.

Suggestions For Safe Swallowing

See Appendix B for a more complete set of suggestions that can help your loved one swallow more safely. They encompass the following:

- their mental and physical state
- the setting for meals
- positioning during and after meals
- choosing suitable foods
- taking medication comfortably and safely
- encouraging safe swallowing strategies

Diet Modification

A change in the diet can be an important part of the treatment plan. It is, however, something that people may fear. But if you understand why it is necessary for safety at this time, you can explain this to your loved one and others involved in providing care.

Let's say, for example, your aunt has been found to aspirate "thin" liquids such as juice or tea and this has led to two episodes of pneumonia. Liquids are characterized as *thin* (like water, tea, coffee, or apple juice), *nectar-thick* (like eggnog or tomato juice), *honey-thick* (like a thick cream soup), and *pudding-thick* (as with pureed fruits and vegetables or mashed potatoes with gravy).

In cases where thin liquids present a swallowing problem, they can be mixed with a taste-free thickener. The thickener can allow for greater control in swallowing, which may reduce the risk of aspiration.

Thickening agents or prepared drinks are readily available through your local pharmacy or online providers. Because thickeners are considered a medical food, check online for side effects (FDA. gov), with your doctor, and with your SLP before you use them.

When a person is on thickened liquids, it is more important than ever to watch out for dehydration because it can be difficult to achieve adequate daily fluid intake by mouth.

Changing the texture of *solid foods*, too, can make swallowing safer. Softer foods place fewer demands upon jaw muscles that are weak or tire easily. Ground food, tofu, and pudding will be easier to chew when dentures are loose-fitting or painful and may be kinder to inflamed cheek and gum tissues.

There is a great deal of nuance in implementing dietary modifications (for example, in selecting suitable foods and in using thickening agents). So, tap into your SLP's knowledge and experience.

It Can Get Emotional

People don't like to hear about changes in their diet. They often feel that something precious is being taken away from them.

We understand. At this point they may have lost many of their most pleasurable habits and routines. When a change in diet is recommended, they may respond with fear, anger, or denial and refuse the new diet.

For now, however, the change may be required for safety—to prevent choking and aspiration—while maintaining nutrition and hydration.

The change in diet may not be permanent. That will depend upon your particular swallowing problem and response to treatment. For those who require a modified diet, they should know there's plenty of delicious, healthy food available. See our **Index** under *recipes*.

"Nothing By Mouth"

At times it may be necessary to bypass swallowing altogether to reduce the risk of choking or aspiration. After a stroke, for example, a person may be made

"NPO" (Latin for *nil per os*). That means they are not allowed to take anything by mouth.

For short-term use, say, thirty days or less, a *nasogastric tube* extending from nose to stomach may be used for feeding. For longer periods, the feeding tube may be placed directly into the stomach. One such tube, inserted by means of percutaneous endoscopic gastrostomy, is often referred to as a *PEG-tube*.

The Risk of Aspiration Remains

Keep in mind that even with tube feeding a person can aspirate. Recall that aspiration of bacteria-laden saliva can lead to pneumonia—hence, the importance of intensive oral care (see below).

Diet modification and tube feeding can serve as a *bridge to the future*—a future with a functional, relatively safe swallow. Many stroke patients, for example, will be able to resume eating a normal diet within several weeks to a few months. So, be patient. Follow the treatment plan.

While healing and therapy are underway, your understanding and support as a loving caregiver can help prevent dangerous slip-ups. Make sure your family knows, as you do, why sneaking a cheeseburger to Uncle Billy for his birthday—while he's recovering from a stroke—will not be doing him a favor. It could cost him his life.

What About Water?

For a person who has difficulty swallowing water, should water be thickened?

This is a complex issue. There are, broadly speaking, two approaches. One approach does indeed recommend thickening the water. The other approach recommends keeping the water as it is—while thickening other liquids. The latter approach (permitting "unthickened" water) carries with it an increased risk of aspiration—with possible complications of pneumonia and death.

The ultimate choice between these approaches (and others) will be based upon assessment of safety factors combined with an individual's wishes. Once again, this is an area that calls for careful assessment of risks versus benefits with close communication between professionals and the patient and family.

Mealtime Strategies

Involve the person you are caring for in preparing food. This can stimulate the appetite and promote saliva flow, which we know is a good thing.

Allow plenty of time for eating. A caregiver must realize that paying too much attention to the clock can invite aspiration or choking.

Eat a small amount at a time. Never has it been more true that you shouldn't bite off more than you can chew.

Chew thoroughly. We're not suggesting that you or your aunt count the number of chews. But we do recommend chewing until the food becomes soft, pasty, and easy to swallow.

Don't talk and eat at the same time. Talking is intimately connected with breathing. When you're excited about sharing something that's on your mind, it's easy to forget you have food or liquid in your mouth. So hold onto that thought and share it after a successful swallow.

Make sure you complete one swallow before you begin another. After you swallow, make sure there's nothing left behind. A caregiver may need to sweep the pockets between cheek and gum with a finger or swab to assure that nothing is left over that can be aspirated.

Alternate solids with liquids to moisten the mouth and throat. This helps move the bolus along and washes away food remnants in the mouth and throat, minimizing the risk of aspiration.

Between swallows, clear the throat with a gentle cough, then swallow again. This helps remove food residue in the throat. Repeat as needed.

Arrange for smaller, more frequent meals. This may enhance safe swallowing when weakness, fatigue, or shortness of breath reduces the effectiveness of swallowing muscles. A person who eats with vigor at the start of a meal may tire as the meal progresses. Muscle fatigue increases the risk of aspiration or choking.

Sip—Don't Guzzle or Gulp

As discussed in Chapter 3, drinking from a cup can be a challenge for many, especially for persons who breathe through their mouth. Breathing stops for several seconds, which can create anxiety that increases the risk of aspiration.

Taking in a large amount of liquid at one time—gulping, guzzling, or chugging—can be risky for anyone with a swallowing problem. (Even without an identified swallowing problem, a person can be surprised by a large volume of liquid suddenly delivered by a wide-mouthed water bottle.) So, for the sake of safety as well as enjoyment, take it one manageable sip at a time.

Using a straw can help, too. But take care—especially in persons with respiratory disease. A large squirt of liquid that arrives unexpectedly at the throat can readily be aspirated. Flexible straws allow for greater control. Be sure the straw is not too far back in the mouth and keep the sips small. Your SLP will guide you as to using (or avoiding) straws.

As mentioned in Chapter 6, specially designed cups can deliver a small, fixed amount of liquid per swallow.

Be On The Lookout

At all times, watch for signs of distress (such as choking, coughing, tearing, or regurgitation through the nose). Be ready to carry out the Heimlich maneuver, if necessary, for choking on food, medication, or other (solid) object (see Chapter 4). Watch the Adam's apple. Does it go up and forward with the swallow? If it doesn't, be suspicious that the swallow was ineffective. Food may remain in the mouth or throat.

Be aware, however, that movement of the Adam's apple does not by itself mean that a safe, effective swallow has occurred.

Don't reload the fork or spoon until you're sure that a successful swallow has been completed. You may need to sweep your mouth with your tongue (or, for a caregiver, with finger or swab). Remember—no food should be left behind.

Swallowing Therapies

The swallowing therapist may call into play positioning techniques, specific swallowing maneuvers, or therapeutic exercises to improve your swallow. One such positioning technique is the *chin tuck*, also called the *chin-down posture*. This involves tucking your chin to your chest while swallowing. The therapist may assist with a gentle touch to the head.

Turning your head to the side during the swallow is another positioning technique. With stroke patients and others this position uses the stronger side to move food or liquid safely from mouth to throat to esophagus while protecting the airway.

The *effortful swallow* is an example of a swallowing maneuver. The patient is asked to swallow with effort, to "swallow hard." This facilitates the oral and pharyngeal phases of swallowing. (See Chapter 6, p. 91.) Repetition of effortful swallowing can make swallowing muscles stronger.

Positioning techniques and swallowing maneuvers may be used singly or in combination, depending upon the particulars of your swallowing situation. Keep in mind that as your swallow becomes safer, these postures and maneuvers may no longer be necessary.

Exercises for Swallowing

Exercising *swallowing muscles* of the face, tongue, lips, cheeks, throat, and larynx can build strength and endurance while enhancing speed and mobility. Working on your *respiratory (chest) muscles*, too, can help you swallow more safely by improving the coordination between your breathing and swallowing and making your protective cough stronger.

Your therapist may have you use a handheld device to blow into forcefully—an *expiratory muscle strength trainer (EMST)*. This has been found to improve swallow safety in persons with Parkinson disease, reducing aspiration and penetration. Other devices have been developed to strengthen the tongue and increase intraoral pressure.

The upper esophageal sphincter can also benefit from exercise. Lying flat and elevating the head according to the Shaker ("shah-KAIR") exercise protocol can extend the time the UES stays open. That promotes a safer, more complete passage of the bolus.

Your therapist will choose the exercises best suited to your needs.

Goals of Swallowing Exercises

- To close the airway at the level of the vocal folds (larynx)
- To improve ability to clear residue in the pharynx
- To strengthen tongue base function
- To increase pressure generation
- To maximize forward and upward movement of the larynx
- To increase opening of the UES
- To strengthen neck muscles
- To maximize chewing, manipulation, and control of the bolus

More on Exercise

A person's medical or neurologic condition may influence their ability to participate in and benefit from a program of swallowing exercises. Persons with congestive heart failure, myasthenia gravis, multiple sclerosis, or ALS, for example, fatigue easily.

In other circumstances, exercise-induced changes in pulse, blood pressure, or respiratory function may preclude some exercises entirely.

Participating in an exercise program requires understanding, attention, and motivation. So persons with cognitive or language limitations, such as those with dementia, stroke, or brain injury, may require cognitive as well as swallowing therapy.

Once the speech-language pathologist has developed a suitable exercise program, she or he can instruct the patient, family members, and other caregivers as to how to carry out this part of the treatment plan.

Keep in mind that although this form of treatment does not involve medication or surgery, exercises related to swallowing may be *very helpful* in establishing a safer swallow.

Sensory Stimulation

The swallowing reflex depends upon sensation: the ability to feel. If the throat is unable to detect the presence of food, the swallowing reflex will be delayed or not triggered at all. As a result, food can remain dangerously behind and put a person at risk of choking or aspiration.

To enhance the sensory component of the swallowing reflex, the therapist may employ techniques of stimulating the throat by thermal or other means. This can be done, for example, with an ice-cold cotton-tipped applicator dipped in lemon juice to activate the swallowing reflex. In some cases, the therapist will stimulate the throat with carbonated beverages.

Stimulating the sense of smell, too, can improve the swallowing reflex. And stimulating the gums as part of an oral care program can increase tactile input needed for swallowing.

Electrical Stimulation

Electrical stimulation has been used and is being investigated in the treatment of swallowing problems. The results to date are inconclusive.

Some of the treatments involve stimulation of swallowing structures of the throat by means of electrodes applied to the skin. Other techniques directly stimulate the inner surface of the mouth and throat. The goal is to improve swallowing by enhancing muscle function, sensory elements of swallowing, or both.

Before pursuing treatment with electrical stimulation, discuss this treatment option carefully with your doctor and swallowing specialist as to contraindications and the likelihood of benefit versus side effects.

Prostheses and Surgery

In some persons with head and neck cancer, a prosthetic soft palate can be designed to prevent nasal regurgitation. In stroke patients with paralysis of the soft palate, surgical attachment of the paralyzed part to the throat can likewise reduce nasal regurgitation and lessen the risk of aspiration.

Injection of botulinum toxin into saliva-producing parotid and submandibular glands may be used to treat drooling (as with ALS). Injection into the lower esophageal sphincter (in treating achalasia) can cause the LES to relax. These effects are temporary, lasting up to several months. Hence, injections may need to be repeated.

Dilation of the esophagus may be carried out to widen narrowing caused by scarring that has resulted from chronic reflux. Depending upon a person's symptoms, surgery may be undertaken for a Zenker diverticulum.

Keep in mind that after surgery, it may still be necessary to maintain other aspects of the treatment plan such as postural techniques, swallowing maneuvers, and modification of the diet.

Oral Care Counts!

The mouth (which includes the tongue, teeth, gums, cheeks, palate, and dentures) provides a rich environment for germs that can be aspirated to cause life-threatening pneumonia. These bacteria can also get into the bloodstream to cause infection of the heart, brain, bones, and joints.

That's why a regular program of oral care—three times a day, after every meal—is important. For those with an impaired immune system (as with cancer or HIV/AIDS) or a chronic medical illness (such as congestive heart failure or COPD), a more intensive oral care program—every 2 to 4 hours— may be required.

Since saliva is an important immunologic "defender" of the oral cavity, persons with *xerostomia* (dry mouth) are at especially high risk of bacterial illness stemming from inadequate oral care. Leading causes of xerostomia are (1) medications (especially anticholinergic agents), (2) Sjögren's syndrome, and (3) head and neck radiation.

Your Oral Care Program

Oral care includes the use of a toothbrush (manual or electric) for teeth and dentures; swabs to moisturize and soothe the lips, tongue, and cheeks; alcohol-free mouth rinses containing antibacterial agents; and (when indicated) suctioning of pooled saliva, which can be teeming with bacteria.

Dentures require special mention. Poorly-fitting dentures can injure underlying gum tissue, making it susceptible to local infection. Painful dentures can dangerously interfere with adequate chewing. Tightly-fitting dentures can trap bacteria. Keep in mind when you're cleaning your dentures, don't forget to clean your mouth as well.

If a patient is NPO, receiving nutrition via tube-feeding, regular oral care is a must, as the mouth remains a fertile site for growth of bacteria.

The oral care program should be combined with regular dental visits and professional cleanings.

Not all suggestions will apply to everyone. Highlight those you consider most useful or copy them onto another sheet of paper. Check with your swallowing specialist as to what best suits your loved one. Post your list on the refrigerator and share with other caregivers.

Ongoing Evaluation and Treatment

The swallowing specialist will follow your progress to see what is working, what is not, and address any new problems that may have arisen. She may arrange for further testing, referral for additional evaluation, or changes in your diet.

Be sure to keep the doctor, nurse, and swallowing specialist informed as to advance directives (including decisions as to tube feeding and do not resuscitate orders) and changes in your loved one's condition. If you think the treatment plan is not working, let them know as soon as possible.

The Treatment Plan

- Understanding the problem
- The setting
- Positioning
- Food choices
- Postural techniques
- Swallowing maneuvers
- Diet modification
- Sensory stimulation
- Oral care
- Minimizing medication side effects
- Prostheses or surgical procedures
- Followup examination and re-evaluation

Challenges For Patient and Caregivers

Some of you reading this book are facing complicated, wrenching, quality-of-life and end-of-life issues. Because swallowing is so closely related to nutrition and hydration and associated with dangers of choking, aspiration, and pneumonia, it often becomes a focus of decision-making in these critical situations.

Issues might include tube-feeding, intravenous hydration, or diet modification. The speech-language pathologist can play a crucial role in bringing key information to the patient and family in a hospital, hospice, or palliative care setting.

The SLP will teach you about pros and cons of each treatment option. You will be the one to make the final decision with family support as needed.

Accepting or Rejecting a Recommendation

Once a swallowing problem has been recognized and a treatment plan developed, the patient (or suitably-designated decision-maker) may wish to pursue a course of action that differs from that recommended by the swallowing specialist or team.

Take for example a woman who, after several bouts of pneumonia, was found to aspirate thin liquids. Aspiration was diagnosed on the basis of bedside examination confirmed by a modified barium swallow. Thickened liquids were recommended to lessen the risk of aspiration.

She tried to drink her beloved coffee, now thickened, but couldn't stand the texture. "I'm not drinking that!" she stated firmly.

She understood that she had a swallowing problem—a tendency to aspirate—and that choosing to continue to drink coffee her way could lead to more pneumonia with a potentially fatal outcome.

She discussed the matter with her family and her swallowing specialist. To make things as clear as possible, she wrote down her thoughts, feelings, desires, and intentions.

Understanding the risks, she chose to continue to drink her coffee "undoctored"—without any thickener. She would do so as safely as possible. For her, that meant sipping slowly, tucking chin to chest while swallowing, clearing her throat after the swallow, and swallowing again before taking another sip.

A patient who rejects the recommendation of the swallowing specialist or the swallowing team can present a dilemma for physicians, nurses, and therapists committed to ethical principles of their professions while respecting the position of the patient and family.

In such situations, it may be valuable to involve a social worker, psychologist, psychiatrist, elder care lawyer, priest, minister, rabbi, or other member of the clergy to help clarify matters.

An Advance Directive

The individual and family may choose a health care proxy to make health care decisions on behalf of a person should he or she become incapacitated. An *advance medical directive* (such as a living will) might specify, for example, that changes in texture of food or liquid would be allowed but not tube feeding of any kind.

Seeing to it that the wishes of your loved one are dealt with in a manner most appropriate for him or her can reduce everyone's anxiety and allow for the fullest remaining life experience.

Communication Is Crucial

The care of the dying patient is complex. The goals of treatment often change, for example, from cure to comfort care.

The cognitive state may decline: from awareness and active participation in treatment to confusion and refusal. Basic medical needs may shift. For hydration, the goals may be limited to alleviating thirst and keeping the mouth comfortably moist. In fact, it has been suggested that a degree of dehydration may bring comfort to a dying person by promoting release of natural pain-relieving substances.

Loss of appetite may itself be a sign that the physical self is winding down. Knowing that, family members may be better able to deal with their loved one's refusal of food, which throughout life has been such an important symbol of wellbeing and nurturance.

Now perhaps more than ever, communication between the dying person, his or her family, members of the clergy, the social worker, and the medical team (primary physician, medical specialists, speech-language pathologist, dietitian, and others) is of especial importance in maximizing choice, dignity, respect, self-determination, and quality of life.

Your Crucial Role as Caregiver

Throughout the diagnostic and therapeutic process, keep in mind the unique and vital role you play—as spouse, child, friend, or professional caregiver.

What you observe in the hospital, at home, or at a care center provides the physician and swallowing specialist with important information they are not able to gain directly.

You help your loved one understand what the problems are and what to do about them.

Your caring ensures that recommendations are carried out to a reasonable and safe degree.

You help prepare nutritious and tasty meals that are best suited to their needs.

You help your loved one use safe swallowing strategies—keeping in mind that choking remains a danger as long as anything is taken by mouth.

You help them practice their exercises.

You help them take their pills comfortably and safely.

You help them reduce the risk of choking, aspiration, dehydration, and malnutrition.

Your love guides you to learn more.

You help establish and maintain a safe and respectful environment for your loved one.

Your patience and strength enable you to be with someone you love through difficult times.

You are the glue that holds it all together.

CHAPTER 9

MINDFUL SWALLOW, SAFE SWALLOW

MINDFUL SWALLOW, SAFE SWALLOW

We hope that by now you've developed a feel for swallowing problems and what to do about them.

Keep learning. Don't stop observing or asking questions. Be prepared at all times for a choking emergency. If and when you do encounter a problem or have a concern, take action. Don't wait for it to go away.

We realize there's no absolute way to protect everyone from every swallowing problem. We feel, though, that knowing how swallowing works and how things can go wrong, you are in a good position to recognize, deal with, and prevent swallowing problems that could affect an elderly person, a younger adult with a medical or neurologic disorder, your children, or yourself.

Attention, Boomers!

Many of you reading this book are Baby Boomers— between the ages of about 45 and 65—participating in the care of an ill elderly parent, a spouse, or an adult child. Share this book with them and with others involved in their care.

You can do a few simple things to help your loved ones stay out of harm's way. Remind them about the importance of not rushing through meals, eating food in small bites, chewing well, finishing a swallow before speaking, and other things you've learned in this book.

Be aware of side effects of medication upon swallowing. Regularly review with the prescribing doctor medications you or your loved one are taking. Eliminate those that are no longer needed or whose side effects outweigh the benefits.

If you suspect a swallowing problem, don't delay in getting help. As you know, something as subtle as frequent throat-clearing during meals, teary eyes, or a voice change afterwards can indicate a swallowing problem. (It may be the presenting symptom of an undiagnosed illness.) The next incident might be a fatal choking episode or a bout of aspiration pneumonia that puts your mother or father into the hospital never to return.

Contact your primary medical provider as soon as possible. Use the *Letter For Your Doctor* to record your observations and concerns.

Do not, however, simply hand off the *Letter* and turn your back on the situation. Continue to be on the alert for the often-subtle symptoms of swallowing difficulty. Maintain safe swallowing strategies and stay in touch with the doctor and therapist.

Day To Day With Your Family

As you sit down at mealtimes with your family, take pleasure in the setting and the company. Enhance your relationship with your spouse. Develop a stronger bond with your children.

Eating breakfast while watching TV and checking your e-mail is all too common these days. Nothing gets your full attention. Little good can come from that. Save your multitasking for later.

If you are mindful while eating—engaged in the present—you will likely enjoy your food more, appreciate its nutritional value, chew it better, cut down on overeating, and reduce the chance of a swallowing mishap.

When it comes to celebrating at home or in a restaurant, be aware that risks can be multiplied. Talking, laughing, drinking alcohol, and swallowing make for a dangerous combination.

So, slow down. Take a breath. Relax. Smell your food. Taste it. Chew thoroughly. Feel the food change from solid to soft.

Enjoy the process. Celebrate this wonderful aspect of life. And....**SWALLOW SAFELY!**

APPENDIX A

LETTER FOR YOUR DOCTOR

Appendix A: Letter For Your Doctor

Date_____

Dear Doctor_____

I am concerned about swallowing in

_____   _____
Name of Person   Date of Birth

She/He is my   Mother   Father   Wife   Husband

other _____

I have noticed these problems over the past:

_____ weeks _____months. *Circle those that apply*:

difficulty swallowing   coughing   choking   gagging

wheezing   teary eyes   runny nose   chest pain

nasal regurgitation   weight loss   recurrent fevers

hurts to swallow   sore throat   refuses food   drooling

voice change: hoarse   weak   gurgly   nasal

frequent throat-clearing   tired out by eating   nausea

loss of taste or smell   bites tongue   burps frequently

food feels stuck/won't go down   food sticks to throat

difficulty with: juice   meat   pills   other _____

embarrassed to eat in public   favorite foods

eats very slowly   tired out by eating   struggles to eat

eats rapidly   dehydration   sore gums   loose dentures

bad breath   recent fall   gets dizzy with swallowing

other observations_____

From SWALLOW SAFELY www.swallowsafely.com

SWALLOW SAFELY

She/He has these medical problems:

_____

_____

_____

Her/His last hospitalization was _____ (date)

at _____(hospital)

for these reasons:_____

_____

She/He is taking the following medications

(prescribed and over-the-counter):

_____

_____

_____

I am most concerned about: choking   aspiration

pneumonia   nutrition   hydration

difficulty swallowing pills

Other_____

_____

From SWALLOW SAFELY   www.swallowsafely.com

Appendix A: Letter For Your Doctor

I look forward to hearing from you at your earliest convenience.

You can reach me in the following ways:

Home Phone ( )_____

Cell Phone ( )_____

E-Mail _____

Fax ( )_____

Mailing Address _____

_____

Thank you very much for your attention and concern.

Sincerely,

_____
Your signature

_____
Your name printed

APPENDIX B

SUGGESTIONS FOR SAFE SWALLOWING

Suggestions
For Safe Swallowing

MENTAL AND PHYSICAL STATE

- Don't eat if drowsy, confused, or agitated.
- Don't eat if unusually weak or out of breath.

SETTING

- Reduce distractions: Turn off TV, radio, cell phone.
- Relaxing music is OK.
- Close doors to reduce traffic.
- Don't overdo conversation or promote laughter while eating.

POSITIONING

- Sit upright, not tilted back or slumped to the side.
- Provide firm support for legs.

FOOD PREPARATION

- Involve the person with a swallowing problem in preparing food to promote saliva flow and overall enthusiasm for eating.
- Check temperature of food and liquids to make sure they are not excessively hot or annoyingly cold.
- Avoid difficult-to-swallow foods such as crusty bread, toast, popcorn, raw vegetables (such as celery or lettuce), whole nuts, and peanut butter.

- Avoid crumbly, flaky foods and pastries dusted with sugar.
- Be careful with (or avoid altogether) carbonated beverages unless otherwise directed.
- Watch out for foods of mixed consistency such as some fruit and cereal with milk.
- Be careful with foods (like ice cream or Jello) that melt.
- Avoid foods or liquids that have caused prior difficulty.
- Provide tasty foods of suitable consistency.
- Thicken liquids as directed.

MEALTIME STRATEGIES

- Don't rush.
- Eat a small amount at a time.
- Chew thoroughly.
- Don't talk and eat at the same time.
- Use the chin tuck maneuver, as directed.
- Swallow, clear throat with a gentle cough, and swallow again before taking in more food.
- Finish the swallow before reloading spoon or fork.
- After the swallow, check mouth for left-over food or pill.
- Clear the mouth, if needed, by tongue, hand, or mechanical suction.
- Alternate solids and liquids to facilitate passage of the bolus and wash away residue.
- Watch for fatigue; finish meal another time, if necessary.
- Arrange for smaller, more frequent meals.
- Note cough, sputter, choke, gag, tearing, runny nose, nasal regurgitation, or voice change.
- If someone coughs or chokes, do not slap on the back.
- Be prepared to carry out the Heimlich maneuver.
- If a choking person leaves the room, *follow him or her.*
- Stay with the person until the incident is resolved.

TAKING MEDICATION

- Stay calm.
- Sit upright.
- Take one pill at a time.
- Swallow pills with plenty of liquid to make swallowing easier and to protect the esophagus.
- Don't exceed daily fluid requirements.
- Use applesauce to facilitate pill-taking.
- Replace difficult-to-swallow pills with more suitable preparations, as approved by a pharmacist.
- Use a specialized cup, if allowed.
- Take medications as early in the day as possible.
- Remain upright for 30 minutes after taking pills.
- In general, use the same strategies that work for swallowing solids and liquids (e.g., effortful swallow, chin tuck).

AFTER MEALS

- Do not lie down for 30-45 minutes after eating.
- Walk for several minutes if permitted.
- Clean teeth, gums, and dentures several times per day.
- Use an antibacterial mouth rinse as prescribed.
- Swab lips, tongue, and cheeks to moisturize and lubricate the mouth.
- Suction pooled saliva to reduce the bacterial load.
- Arrange for regular dental care.

BETWEEN MEALS

- Watch for respiratory difficulty (such as cough, rapid breathing, or wheezing), chest pain, or voice change.
- Carry out approved swallowing-related exercises that involve breathing, coughing, and chewing.

- Work on overall fitness, muscle strength, balance, and posture.
- Keep mind and body active with reading, playing bridge and Scrabble, doing word puzzles and Sudoku, mentoring, and other activities (such as brain-training exercises).
- At bedtime, elevate the head of bed to 30 degrees to help prevent aspiration or reflux during sleep.

Appendix C

Anticholinergic Drugs by Category

ANTICHOLINERGIC DRUGS
BY CATEGORY

Antihistamines
chlorpheniramine	Chlor-Trimeton, Polaramine
cyproheptadine	Periactin
dimenhydrinate	Dramamine
diphenhydramine	Benadryl, Compoz, Nytol, Unisom
hydroxyzine	Atarax, Vistaril
promethazine	Phenergan

Antiparkinsonian
benztropine	Cogentin
procyclidine	Kemadrin
trihexyphenidyl	Artane

Antivertigo
meclizine	Antivert
prochlorperazine	Compazine
promethazine	Phenergan

Cardiac
disopyramide	Norpace
procainamide	Procanbid
quinidine	Cardioquin, Quinidex, Quinora

Gastrointestinal

belladonna preparations (containing atropine, hyoscine, hyoscyamine, or scopolamine)	Donnatal (includes phenobarbital)
glycopyrrolate	Robinul
hyoscyamine	Levsin
propantheline	Pro-Banthine
dicyclomine	Bentyl

Herbal Preparations

Atropa belladonna (deadly nightshade)
Brugmansia species (Angel's trumpet)
Datura stramonium (datura)
Hyoscyamus niger (henbane)
Mandragora officinarum (mandrake)

Psychiatric

Major Tranquilizers/Antipsychotics

chlorpromazine	Thorazine
clozapine	Clozaril
fluphenazine	Prolixin
haloperidol	Haldol
perphenazine	Trilafon
thioridazine	Mellaril
thiothixene	Navane

Antidepressants

amitriptyline	Elavil
clomipramine	Anafranil
desipramine	Norpramine

imipramine	Tofranil
nortriptyline	Aventyl, Pamelor
doxepin	Sinequan

Respiratory

| *ipratropium* | Atrovent |
| *tiotropium* | Spiriva |

Skeletal Muscle Relaxants

cylcobenzaprine	Flexeril
dantrolene	Dantrium
methocarbamol	Robaxin
orphenadrine	Norflex

Urinary Tract

| *oxybutynin* | Ditropan |
| *tolterodine* | Detrol |

REFERENCES

Chapter 1. Why We Wrote This Book

Altman KW, Yu G-P, Schaefer SD: Consequence of Dysphagia in the Hospitalized Patient. Impact on Prognosis and Hospital Resources. *Arch Otolaryngol Head and Neck Surg* (2010) 136:784-89.

Boyce JM, Potter-Bynoe G, Dziobek L, RN; Solomon SL: Nosocomial pneumonia in Medicare patients: Hospital costs and reimbursement patterns under the prospective payment system. *Archives of Internal Medicine* (1991) 151:1109-14.

Carpenter S: Treating an illness is one thing. What about a patient with many? *The New York Times*, March 31, 2009. http://www.nytimes.com/2009/03/31/health/31sick.html

Centers for Disease Control and Prevention (CDC): Important Facts About Falls. Updated Jan. 20, 2016. http://www.cdc.gov/homeandrecreationalsafety/falls/adultfalls.html. *See also*, https://www.nia.nih.gov/health/publication/falls-and-fractures

Evans, C: Malnutrition in the elderly: A multifactorial failure to thrive. *Permanente Journal* (2005) 9:38-41.

Gorard DA: Escalating polypharmacy. *Quarterly Journal of Medicine* (2006) 99:797-800.

H.Con.Res. 195 - 110th Congress (2007-08): National Dysphagia Awareness Month. *See also*, http://swallowingdisorderfoundation.com/awareness/

Katzan IL, Dawson NV, Thomas CL, Votruba ME, Cebul RD: The cost of pneumonia after acute stroke. *Neurology* (2007) 68:1938-43.

Kramarow E, Chen LH, Hedegaard H, Warner M: Deaths from unintentional injury among adults aged 65 and over: United States, 2000–2013. NCHS data brief, no. 199. Hyattsville, MD: National Center for Health Statistics. 2015.

165

Murry T, Carrau RL, Eibling DE: "Epidemiology of Swallowing Disorders," Chapter 1, in *Comprehensive Management of Swallowing Disorders*, Carrau RL, Murry T (eds.), Singular Publishing Group, Inc., San Diego, CA, 1999, pp. 3-7.

National Center for Health Statistics: Accidents or Unintentional Injuries: Unintentional fall deaths. Updated Sep. 30, 2015.

Perkins-Carpenter B: *How To Prevent Falls: Better Balance, Independence and Energy in 6 Simple Steps*. Senior Fitness Productions, Inc., Penfield, NY, 2006.

Robbins JA, Banaszynski K: "Swallowing Problems in Older Adults." Chapter 9, in *Geriatric Nutrition, 4th Ed.*, Chernoff R (ed.), Jones & Bartlett Learning, Burlington, MA, 2014, pp. 211-12.

Sharp HM, Bryant KN: Ethical issues in dysphagia: When patients refuse assessment or treatment. *Seminars in Speech and Language* (2003) 24:285-99.

Tinetti ME, Kumar C: The patient who falls: "It's always a trade-off." *Journal of the American Medical Association* (2010) 303:258-266.

Winakur J: What are we going to do with Dad? A geriatrician stands by during his father's downward spiral into old age, disability, and dementia. *Health Affairs* (2005) 24:1064-1072.

Chapter 2. How Swallowing Works

Aviv JE: "The Normal Swallow," Chapter 3, in *Comprehensive Management of Swallowing Disorders*, Carrau RL, Murry T (eds.), Singular Publishing Group, Inc., San Diego, CA, 1999, pp. 23-29.

Linkinhoker M: "Swallowing, An Animated Sequence." Johns Hopkins Medicine Health Library: Swallowing Disorders, 2002. *See also*, http://linkstudio.info/company/

Logemann JA: "Anatomy and Physiology of Normal Deglutition." Chapter 2, in *Evaluation and Treatment of Swallowing Disorders, 2nd ed.*, PRO-ED, Inc., Austin, TX, 1998, pp. 13-35.

Martin-Harris B, Brodsky MB, Michel Y, Ford CL, Walters B, Heffner J: Breathing and swallowing dynamics across the adult lifespan. *Archives of Otolaryngology—Head and Neck Surgery* (2005) 131:762-70.

References

Shune SE, Moon JB, Goodman SS: The effects of age and pre-oral sensorimotor cues on anticipatory mouth movement during swallowing. *Journal of Speech, Language, and Hearing Research,* March 2016.

Chapter 3. When Swallowing Doesn't Work

Abraham S, Scheinberg LC, Smith CR, LaRocca NG: Neurologic Impairment and Disability Status in Outpatients with Multiple Sclerosis Reporting Dysphagia Symptomatology. *Neurorehabil Neural Repair* (1997) 11:7-13.

American Speech-Language-Hearing Association (ASHA): "Swallowing Disorders (Dysphagia) in Adults."

Aslam M, Vaezi MF: Dysphagia in the Elderly. *Gastroenterology & Hepatology* (2013) 9:784-95.

Bedore B: Management of Dysphagia in Individuals with Amyotrophic Lateral Sclerosis. *Perspectives on Swallowing and Swallowing Disorders (Dysphagia)* (2013) 22:26-31.

Castrogiovanni A: Communication facts: Special populations: Dysphagia–2008 edition. American Speech-Language-Hearing Association.

Brody JE: "When swallowing food becomes a problem." *New York Times,* July 20, 2004.

Carl LL, Johnson PR: "Medications Affecting Appetite, Taste, or Smell." Chapter 12, in *Drugs and Dysphagia: How Medications Can Affect Eating and Swallowing.* PRO-ED, Inc., Austin, TX, 2006, pp. 219-36.

Carrau RL, Murry T: Pathophysiology of Swallowing Disorders. Part IV, in *Comprehensive Management of Swallowing Disorders,* Carrau RL, Murry T (eds.), Singular Publishing Group, Inc., San Diego, CA, 1999, pp. 91-233.

Chaw E, Shem K, Castillo K, Wong SL, Chang J: Dysphagia and Associated Respiratory Considerations in Cervical Spinal Cord Injury. *Topics in Spinal Cord Rehabilitation Injury* (2012) 18:291-99.

Ciucci MR, Grant LM, Rajamanickam ESP, Hilby BL, Blue KV, Jones CA, Kelm-Nelson CA: Early Identification and Treatment of

Communication and Swallowing Deficits in Parkinson Disease. *Semin Speech Lang* (2013) 34:185-202.

Da Silva-Junior FP, Carrasco AEAB, Da Silva Mendes AM, Lopes AJT, Souza, MANE, De Bruin VMS: Swallowing dysfunction in Wilson's disease: A scintigraphic study. *Neurogastroenterol Motil* (2008) 20:285-90.

Edwards D, Bacon E: Optimizing Function for Patients Diagnosed with Cerebral Palsy. *Perspectives on Swallowing and Swallowing Disorders (Dysphagia)* (2014) 23:123-31.

Enzinger PC, Mayer RJ: Esophageal cancer. *New England Journal of Medicine* (2003) 349:2241-52.

Gross RD, Atwood Jr CW, Ross SB, Eichhorn KA, Olszewski JW, Doyle PJ: The coordination of breathing and swallowing in Parkinson's disease. *Dysphagia* (2008) 23:136-45.

Gaude GS: Pulmonary manifestations of gastroesophageal reflux disease. *Ann Thorac Med* (2009) 4:115-23.

Gross RD, Atwood Jr CW, Ross SB, Olszewski JW, Eichhorn KA: The coordination of breathing and swallowing in chronic obstructive pulmonary disease. *American Journal of Respiratory and Critical Care Medicine* (2009) 179:559-65.

Jankovic J: Parkinson's disease: clinical features and diagnosis. *J Neurol Neurosurg Psychiatry* (2008) 79:368-376.

Kazandjian M, Dikeman K: Guillain-Barre Syndrome and Disordered Swallowing. *Perspectives on Swallowing and Swallowing Disorders (Dysphagia)* (2012) 21:115-20.

Kessing BF, Bredenoord AJ, Smout AJ: The pathophysiology, diagnosis and treatment of excessive belching symptoms. *Am J Gastroenterol* (2014) 109:1196-1203.

Khanna S, Noheria A, Rohren CH: 52-Year-Old Woman with Dysphagia. *Mayo Clin Proc* (2010) 85:760-63. *Note*: A case of eosinophilic esophagitis.

Kumar N: "Neurogastroenterology." *Continuum: Lifelong Learning in Neurology* (2008) 14:13-52.

Levy B, Young MA: Pathophysiology of Swallowing and Gastroesophageal Reflux. Chapter 26 in *Comprehensive Management*

References

of Swallowing Disorders, Carrau RL, Murry T (eds.), Singular Publishing Group, Inc., San Diego, CA, 1999, pp. 175-86.

Llabrés M, F J Molina-Martinez FJ, F Miralles F: Dysphagia as the sole manifestation of myasthenia gravis. *J Neurol Neurosurg Psychiatry* (2005) 76:1297-300.

Logemann JA: *Evaluation and Treatment of Swallowing Disorders*, *2nd ed.*, PRO-ED, Inc., Austin, TX, 1998, pp. 1-11, 251-79, 281-306, 307-28, 329-43.

Logemann JA, Curro FA, Pauloski B, Gensler G: Aging effects on oropharyngeal swallow and the role of dental care in oropharyngeal dysphagia. *Oral Dis* (2013) 19:733-37.

Logemann JA, Larsen K: Oropharyngeal dysphagia: pathophysiology and diagnosis for the anniversary issue of *Diseases of the Esophagus*. *Dis. Esophagus* (2012) 25:299-304.

Lundy D, Sullivan P: Xerostomia. *Perspectives on Swallowing and Swallowing Disorders (Dysphagia)* (2012) 21:22-27.

Martino R, Foley N, Bhogal S, Diamant N, Speechley M, Teasell R: Dysphagia after stroke: Incidence, diagnosis, and pulmonary complications. *Stroke* (2005) 36:2756-63.

McCulloch TM, Jaffe D: Head and neck disorders affecting swallowing. *GI Motility Online*, May 16, 2006.

MedlinePlus (National Institutes of Health/U.S. National Library of Medicine): Botulism. Updated March 25, 2016.

Moore PK, Lee JK, Garcia JA, Krantz MJ: A Case of Swallow Syncope. *Tex Heart Inst J* (2013) 40: 606-07.

Murry T, Carrau RL: "The Abnormal Swallow: Conditions and Diseases." Part III, in *Clinical Management of Swallowing Disorders*, *2nd ed.* Plural Publishing, Inc., San Diego, CA, 2006, p, 47.

Nath B, Mahanta TG: Investigation of an Outbreak of Diphtheria in Borborooah Block of Dibrugarh District, Assam. *Indian J Community Med.* (2010) 35:436-38.

Rabenstein AA: Acute Neuromuscular Respiratory Failure. *Continuum* (2015) 21:1324-45.

Ramsey DJC, Smithard DG, Kalra L: Early Assessments of Dysphagia and Aspiration Risk in Acute Stroke Patients. *Stroke* (2003) 34:1252-57.

Saikia L, Nath R, Saikia NJ, Choudhury G, Sarkar M: A diphtheria outbreak in Assam, India. *Southeast Asian J Trop Med Public Health* (2010) 41:647-52.

Sato E, Hirano H, Watanabe Y, Edahiro A, Sato K, Yamane G, Katakura A: Detecting signs of dysphagia in patients with Alzheimer's disease with oral feeding in daily life. *Geriatr Gerontol Int* (2014) 14:549-55.

Schneider SL, Haack L, Owens J, Herrington DP, Zelek A: An Interdisciplinary Treatment Approach for Soldiers with TBI/PTSD: Issues and Outcomes. *Perspectives on Neurophysiology and Neurogenic Speech and Language Disorders* (2009) 19:36-46.

Shastri N, Hogan W: Eosinophilic Esophagitis: The New Kid on the Block. *Perspectives on Swallowing and Swallowing Disorders (Dysphagia)* (2012) 21:43-51.

Sheehan NJ: Dysphagia and other manifestations of oesophageal involvement in the musculoskeletal diseases. *Rheumatology* (2008) 47:746-52.

Stewart C: Dysphagia Symptoms and Treatment in Huntington's Disease: Review. *Perspectives on Swallowing and Swallowing Disorders (Dysphagia)* (2012) 21:126-134.

Sura L, Madhavan A, Carnaby G, Crary MA: Dysphagia in the elderly: management and nutritional considerations. *Clinical Interventions in Aging* (2012) 7:287-98.

Teasell R, Foley N, Martino R, Richardson M, Bhogal S, Speechley M: Dysphagia and Aspiration Following Stroke. *Evidence-Based Review of Stroke Rehabilitation (EBRSR)*, Updated Sept. 2013.

Wilkins T, Gillies RA, Thomas AM, Wagner PJ: The prevalence of dysphagia in primary care patients: A HamesNet research network study. *Journal of the American Board of Family Medicine* (2007) 20:144-50.

Winchester J, Winchester CG: Cognitive Dysphagia and Effectively Managing the Five Systems. *Perspectives on Gerontology* (2015) 20:116-32.

References

Witcik M, Joshua Meskin: Pop and Drop. *WMJ (Wisconsin Medical Journal)* (2014) 113:162-63.

Chapter 4. What To Do About Choking

American Heart Association: "Foreign Body Airway Obstruction (Choking)." In, *2015 AHA Guidelines for CPR & ECC.*

American Red Cross: "Choking." First Aid/CPR/AED. *Participant's Manual.* January 13, 2011, pp. 72-75.

Breatnach E, Abbott GC, Fraser RB: Dimensions of the normal human trachea. *American Journal of Roentgenology* (1984) 141:903-06.

Deaconess Association Incorporated: "How to do the Heimlich maneuver." www.deaconess-healthcare.com/Heimlich_Institute/

Dolkas L, Stanley C, Smith AM, Vilke GM: Deaths associated with choking in San Diego County. *Journal of Forensic Sciences* (2007) 52:176-79.

Ekberg O, Feinberg M: Clinical and demographic data in 75 patients with near-fatal choking episodes. *Dysphagia* (1992) 7:205-08.

Gardner GH *et al.*: American Academy of Pediatrics Policy Statement—Prevention of Choking Among Children. *Pediatrics* (2010) 125:601-07.

Gross RD, Atwood Jr CW, Ross SB, Eichhorn KA, Olszewski JW, Doyle PJ: The coordination of breathing and swallowing in Parkinson's disease. *Dysphagia* (2008) 23:136-45.

Haugen RK: The café coronary: Sudden deaths in restaurants. *JAMA* (1963) 186:142-43.

Heimlich HJ: Pop goes the café coronary. *Emergency Medicine*, June 1974, 154-55.

Heimlich HJ: A Life-Saving Maneuver to Prevent Food-Choking. *JAMA* (1975) 234:398-401.

Heimlich HJ: Albert Lasker Public Service Award: 1984 Winners. http://www.laskerfoundation.org/awards/1984public.htm

Heller JL: Choking First Aid – Adult or Child Over One Year. *MedlinePlus.* Last updated July 20, 2013.

Mittelman RE, Wetli CV: The fatal café coronary: Foreign-body airway obstruction. *JAMA* (1982) 247:1285-88.

Warshawsky ME: Foreign body aspiration. *Medscape.* Updated Dec. 31, 2015.

Wick R, Gilbert JD, Byard RW: Café coronary syndrome – Fatal choking on food: An autopsy approach. *Journal of Clinical Forensic Medicine* (2006) 13:135-38, 2006.

Chapter 5. Aspiration and Pneumonia

American Speech-Language-Hearing Association (ASHA): "Swallowing Disorders (Dysphagia) in Adults."

Argolo N, Sampaio M, Pinho P, Melo A, Nóbrega AC: Videofluoroscopic Predictors of Penetration-Aspiration in Parkinson's Disease Patients. *Dysphagia* (2015) 30:751-58.

Cavallazzi R, Vasu TS, Marik PE: Aspiration Pneumonitis and Aspiration Pneumonia. *Perspectives on Swallowing and Swallowing Disorders (Dysphagia)* (2009) 18:25-33.

Chaw E, Shem K, Castillo K, Wong SL, Chang J: Dysphagia and Associated Respiratory Considerations in Cervical Spinal Cord Injury. *Topics in Spinal Cord Rehabilitation Injury* (2012) 18:291-99.

Ciucci MR, Grant LM, Rajamanickam ESP, Hilby BL, Blue KV, Jones CA, Kelm-Nelson CA: Early Identification and Treatment of Communication and Swallowing Deficits in Parkinson Disease. *Semin Speech Lang* (2013) 34:185-202.

Daniels SK, Brailey K, Priestly DH, Herrington LS, Weisberg LA, Foundas AL: Aspiration in Patients with Acute Stroke. *Arch Phys Med Rehabil* (1998) 79:14-19.

Da Silva-Junior FP, Carrasco AEAB, Da Silva Mendes AM, Lopes AJT, Souza, MANE, De Bruin VMS: Swallowing dysfunction in Wilson's disease: A scintigraphic study. *Neurogastroenterol Motil* (2008) 20:285-90.

Falestiny MN, Yu VL: "Aspiration Pneumonia," Chapter 55 in *Comprehensive Management of Swallowing Disorders*, Carrau RL, Murry T (eds.), Singular Publishing Group, Inc., San Diego, CA, 1999, pp. 383-87.

References

Gaude GS: Pulmonary manifestations of gastroesophageal reflux disease. *Ann Thor Med* (2009) 4:115-23.

Gross RD, Atwood Jr CW, Ross SB, Olszewski JW, Eichhorn KA: The coordination of breathing and swallowing in chronic obstructive pulmonary disease. *Am J Resp Critical Care Med* (2009) 179:559-65.

Heemskerk A-W, Roos RAC: Aspiration pneumonia and death in Huntington's disease. *PLOS Currents*, February 2, 2012.

Huxley EJ, Viroslav J, Gray WR, Pierce AK: Pharyngeal aspiration in normal adults and patients with depressed consciousness. *American Journal of Medicine* (1978) 64:564-68.

Liantonia J, Salzman B, Snyderman D: Preventing Aspiration Pneumonia by Addressing Three Key Risk Factors: Dysphagia, Poor Oral Hygiene, and Medication Use. *Annals of Long Term Care*, October 2014.

Logemann JA: "Introduction: Definitions and Basic Principles of Evaluation and Treatment of Swallowing Disorders," Chapter 1 in *Evaluation and Treatment of Swallowing Disorders, 2nd ed.*, PRO-ED, Inc., Austin, TX, 1998, p. 5.

Marik PE: Aspiration pneumonitis and aspiration pneumonia. *N Engl J Med* (2001) 344:665-71.

Marik PE, Kaplan D: Aspiration pneumonia and dysphagia in the elderly. *Chest* (2003) 124:328-36.

Marks JW: Gastroesophageal reflux disease (GERD, acid reflux, heartburn). *MedicineNet.com*, May 8, 2015.

Martino R, Foley N, Bhogal S, Diamant N, Speechley M, Teasell R: Dysphagia after stroke: Incidence, diagnosis, and pulmonary complications. *Stroke* (2005) 36:2756-63.

Medina-Walpole AM, Katz PR: Nursing home-acquired pneumonia. *J Am Geriatrics Society* (1999) 47:1005-15.

Molfenter SM, Steele CM: The relationship between residue and aspiration on the subsequent swallow: an application of the normalized residue ratio scale. *Dysphagia* (2013) 28:494-500.

Morehead RS: Gastro-oesophageal reflux disease and non-asthma lung disease. *Eur Resp Rev* (2009) 18:233-43.

Ramsey D, Smithard D, Kalra L: Silent aspiration: What do we know? *Dysphagia* (2005) 20:218-25.

Ramsey DJC, Smithard DG, Kalra L: Early Assessments of dysphagia and aspiration risk in acute stroke patients. *Stroke* (2003) 34:1252-57.

Robbins JA, Gensler G, Hind J, Logemann JA, Lindblad AS, Brandt D, Baum H, Lilienfeld D, Kosek S, Lundy D, Dikeman K, Kazandjian M, Gramigna GD, McGarvey-Toler S, Miller Gardner PJ: Comparison of 2 interventions for liquid aspiration on pneumonia incidence: A randomized trial. *Annals of Internal Medicine* (2008) 148:509-18.

Smith Hammond CA, Goldstein LB: Cough and aspiration of food and liquids due to oral-pharyngeal dysphagia. ACCP evidence-based clinical practice guidelines. *Chest* (2006) 129:154S-168S.

Stewart C: Dysphagia Symptoms and Treatment in Huntington's Disease: Review. *Perspectives on Swallowing and Swallowing Disorders (Dysphagia)* (2012) 21:126-134.

Sura L, Madhavan A, Carnaby G, Crary M: Dysphagia in the elderly: management and nutritional considerations. *Clinical Interventions in Aging* (2012) 7:287-98.

Teasell R, Foley N, Martino R, Richardson M, Bhogal S, Speechley M: Dysphagia and Aspiration Following Stroke. *Evidence-Based Review of Stroke Rehabilitation (EBRSR)*, Updated Sept. 2013.

Terpenning M: Geriatric Oral Health and Pneumonia Risk. *Clin Infect Dis* (2005) 40:1807-10.

Troche MS, Okun MS, Rosenbek JC, Musson N, Fernandez HH, Rodriguez R, Romrell J, Pitts T, Wheeler-Hegland KM, Sapienza CM: Aspiration and swallowing in Parkinson disease and rehabilitation with EMST: A randomized trial. *Neurology* (2010) 75:1912-19.

Waito A, Bailey GL, Molfenter SM, Zoratto DC, Steele CM: Voice-quality abnormalities as a sign of dysphagia: validation against acoustic and videofluoroscopic data. *Dysphagia* (2011) 26:125-134.

Warshawsky ME: Foreign body aspiration. *Medscape.* Updated Dec. 31, 2015.

References

Chapter 6. Medication: A Double-Edged Sword

Agarwala SS, Sbeitan I: "Iatrogenic Swallowing Disorders: Chemotherapy." Chapter 18 in *Comprehensive Management of Swallowing Disorders*, Carrau RL, Murry T (eds.), Singular Publishing Group, Inc., San Diego, CA 1999, pp. 124-29.

Alvi A: "Iatrogenic swallowing disorders: Medications." Chapter 17 in *Comprehensive Management of Swallowing Disorders*, Carrau RL, Murry T (eds.), pp. 119-124.

Ancelin ML, Artero S, Portet F, Dupuy A-M, Touchon J, Ritchie K: Non-degenerative mild cognitive impairment in elderly people and use of anticholinergic drugs: longitudinal cohort study. *BMJ* (2006) 332:455-59.

Aparanji KP, Annavarappu S, Russell RO, Dharmarajan TS: Severe Dysphagia from Medication-Induced Esophagitis: A Preventable Disorder. *Clinical Geriatrics*, Vol. 20, February 13, 2012.

Carl L, Johnson P: Drugs and dysphagia. *Perspectives on Swallowing and Swallowing Disorders (Dysphagia)* (2008) 17:143-48.

Carl LL, Johnson PR: "Medications Affecting Appetite, Taste, or Smell." pp. 219-36; "Medications That Cause Esophageal Injury," pp. 261-62, in *Drugs and Dysphagia: How Medications Can Affect Eating and Swallowing*. PRO-ED, Inc., Austin, TX, 2006.

Chatoor I, Conley C, Dickson L. Food refusal after an incident of choking: A posttraumatic eating disorder. *Journal of the American Academy of Child and Adolescent Psychiatry* (1988) 27:105-10.

Couris RR, Gura KM, Blumberg J, Chernoff R: Pharmacology, Nutrition, and Elderly Adults: Interactions and Implications. Chernoff R (Ed.) *Geriatric Nutrition: The Health Professional's Handbook. 4th ed.*, Jones and Bartlett Learning, Burlington, MA, 2013, pp. 377-416

Gosa M: Necrotizing Enterocolitis and the Use of Thickened Liquids for Infants With Dysphagia. *Perspectives on Swallowing and Swallowing Disorders (Dysphagia)* (2015) 24:44-49.

Hajjar ER, Cafiero AC, Hanlon JT: Polypharmacy in elderly patients. *American Journal of Geriatric Pharmacotherapy* (2007) 5:345-51.

Gallagher L: The Impact of Prescribed Medication on Swallowing: An Overview. *Perspectives on Swallowing and Swallowing Disorders (Dysphagia)* (2010) 19:98-102.

Gorard DA: Escalating polypharmacy. *Quarterly Journal of Medicine* (2006) 99:797-800.

Goulding MR: Inappropriate medication prescribing for elderly ambulatory care patients. *Archives of Internal Medicine* (2004) 164:305-12.

Hamilton HJ, Gallagher PF, O'Mahony D: Inappropriate prescribing and adverse drug events in older people. *BioMed Central Geriatrics*, Jan. 28, 2009.

Heidelbaugh JJ: Proton pump inhibitors and risk of vitamin and mineral deficiency: evidence and clinical implications. *Therapeutic Advances in Drug Safety* (2013) 4:125-33.

Jackson LD, Little J, Kung E, Williams EM, Siemiatkowska K, Plowman S: Safe Medication Swallowing in Dysphagia: A Collaborative Improvement Project. *Healthcare Quarterly* (2008) 11:110-16.

Jahromi SR, Togha M, Fesharaki SH, Najafi M, Moghadam NB, Kheradmand JA, Kezemi H, Gorji A: Gastrointestinal adverse effects of antiepileptic drugs in intractable epileptic patients. *Seizure: European Journal of Epilepsy* (2011) 20:343-46.

Jaspersen D: Drug-induced oesophageal disorders: Pathogenesis, incidence, prevention and management. *Drug Safety* (2000) 22:237-49.

Kelly J, Wright D: Administering medication to adult patients with dysphagia. *Nursing Standard* (2009) 23:61-68.

Kikendall JW: Pill-Induced Esophagitis. *Gastroenterology & Hepatology* (N Y) (2007) 3:275-76.

Lagergren J, Bergstrom R, Adami H-O, Nyren O: Association between medications that relax the lower esophageal sphincter and risk for esophageal adenocarcinoma. *Annals of Internal Medicine* (2000) 133:165-75.

MedlinePlus: Drugs, Supplements, and Herbal Information. U.S. National Library of Medicine and National Institutes of Health, Department of Health and Human Services.

References

Mintzer J, Burns A: Anticholinergic side-effects of drugs in elderly people. *Journal of the Royal Society of Medicine* (2000) 93:457-62.

Ruschena D, Mullen PE, Palmer S, Burgess P, Cordner SM, Drummer OH, Wallace C, Barry-Walsh J: Choking deaths: The role of antipsychotic medication. *British Journal of Psychiatry* (2003) 183:446-50.

Seuss D: *You're Only Old Once!* Random House, Inc., New York, NY (1986).

Shapiro J, Franko DL, Gagne A: Phagophobia: A form of psychogenic dysphagia. A new entity. *Annals of Otology, Rhinology and Laryngology* (1997) 106:286-90.

U.S. Food and Drug Administration, U.S. Department of Health and Human Services: www.fda.gov.

Chapter 7. Getting Help

American Speech-Language-Hearing Association (ASHA). "Scope of Practice in Speech-Language Pathology," "End-of-Life Issues in Speech-Language Pathology," "Dysphagia Teams."

Argolo N, Sampaio M, Pinho P, Melo A, Nóbrega AC: Videofluoroscopic Predictors of Penetration-Aspiration in Parkinson's Disease Patients. *Dysphagia* (2015) 30:751-58.

Bours GJ, Speyer R, Lemmens J, Limburg M, de Wit R: Bedside screening tests vs. videofluoroscopy or fibreoptic endoscopic evaluation of swallowing to detect dysphagia in patients with neurological disorders: systematic review. *Journal of Advanced Nursing* (2009) 65:477-93.

Brady S, Donzelli J: The modified barium swallow and the functional endoscopic evaluation of swallowing. *Otolaryngol Clin North Am* (2013) 46:1009-22.

Coyle JL: The Clinical Evaluation: A Necessary Tool for the Dysphagia Sleuth. *Perspectives on Swallowing and Swallowing Disorders (Dysphagia)* (2015) 24:18-25.

Doggett DL, Tappe KA, Mitchell MD, Chapell R, Coates V, Turkelson CM: Prevention of pneumonia in elderly stroke patients by systematic diagnosis and treatment of dysphagia: An evidence-based comprehensive analysis of the literature. *Dysphagia* (2001) 16:279-95.

Easterling C: The Esophagus, To Screen or Not To Screen...That Is the Question, the Responsibility, and Liability. *Perspectives on Swallowing and Swallowing Disorders (Dysphagia)* (2012) 21:68-72.

Hegland K, Sapienza C: SLP's Role in Evaluation and Treatment of Cough Function. *Perspectives on Swallowing and Swallowing Disorders (Dysphagia)* (2013) 22:85-93.

Hinchey JA, Shephard T, Furie K, Smith D, Wang D, Tonn S: Formal dysphagia screening protocols prevent pneumonia. *Stroke* (2005) 36:1972-76.

Langmore S, Murray J: Fiberoptic Endoscopic Evaluation of Swallowing (FEES). In *Manual of Diagnostic and Therapeutic Techniques for Disorders of Deglutition*. Shaker R, Easterling, C, Belafsky PC, Postma GN (eds). Springer, New York, NY, 2012, pp. 85-101.

Leder SB: Comparing Simultaneous Clinical Swallow Evaluations and Fiberoptic Endoscopic Evaluations of Swallowing: Findings and Consequences. *Perspectives on Swallowing and Swallowing Disorders (Dysphagia)* (2015) 24:12-17.

Levine MS: Radiographic Evaluation of the Esophageal Phase of Swallowing. In *Manual of Diagnostic and Therapeutic Techniques for Disorders of Deglutition*. Shaker R, Easterling, C, Belafsky PC, Postma GN (eds). Springer, New York, NY, 2012, pp. 49-84.

Logemann J: "Videofluoroscopy" (pp. 58-61), "Videoendoscopy" (pp. 54-59), "Videofluoroscopic procedure—The modified barium swallow" (pp. 168-85). In *Evaluation and Treatment of Swallowing Disorders, 2nd ed.*, PRO-ED, Inc., Austin, TX, 1998.

Logemann JA: Approach to the Patient with Dysphagia. Ch. 18 in *Practical Neurology, 4th ed.*, Biller J, Lippincott Williams and Wilkins, Philadelphia, PA, 2012, pp. 213-22.

Logemann JA, Larsen K: Radiographic Evaluation of the Oral/ Preparatory and Pharyngeal Phases of Swallowing Including the UES: Comprehensive Modified Barium Swallow Studies. In *Manual of Diagnostic and Therapeutic Techniques for Disorders of*

References

Deglutition. Shaker R, Easterling, C, Belafsky PC, Postma GN (eds). Springer, New York, NY, 2012, pp. 33-47.

Malandraki GA, Johnson S, Robbins JA: Functional Magnetic Resonance Imaging of Swallowing Function: From Neurophysiology to Neuroplasticity. Published online September 7, 2011. Final edited form: *Head Neck* (2011) 33:S14-20.

Murry T, Carrau RL: "Functional Tests of Swallowing." Chapter 12 in *Comprehensive Management of Swallowing Disorders*, Carrau RL, Murry T (eds.), Singular Pub. Group, Inc., San Diego, CA, 1999, pp. 75-79.

Patterson KR: Issues of Capacity and Decision-Making in the Context of Delirium. *Perspectives on Swallowing and Swallowing Disorders (Dysphagia)* (2015) 24:140-45.

Ramsey DJC, Smithard DG, Kalra L: Early assessments of dysphagia and aspiration risk in acute stroke patients. *Stroke* (2003) 34:1252-57.

Riquelme LF: Clinical Swallow Examination (CSE): Can We Talk? *Perspectives on Swallowing and Swallowing Disorders (Dysphagia)* (2015) 24:34-39.

Voyzey G: The Speech-Language Pathologist's Role Assessing Cultural Variations with Patients Receiving Palliative Care. *Perspectives on Gerontology* (2014) 129:100-104.

Waito A, Bailey GL, Molfenter SM, Zoratto DC, Steele CM: Voice-quality abnormalities as a sign of dysphagia: validation against acoustic and videofluoroscopic data. *Dysphagia* (2011) 26:125-134.

Weindling F-H: Speech-language pathology: A home care viewpoint. *Am J Speech Lang Path* (2000) 9:99-106.

Westergren A: Detection of eating difficulties after stroke: A systematic review. *International Nursing Review* (2006) 53:143-49.

Chapter 8. Treating Swallowing Problems

Achilles E: *The Dysphagia Cookbook. Great Tasting and Nutritious Recipes for People with Swallowing Difficulties.* Cumberland House. Nashville, TN, 2004.

ASHA Leader: "International Initiative Standardizes Modified Foods, Thickened Liquids." January 2016.

Ashford JF: Oral Care Across Ages: A Review. *Perspectives on Swallowing and Swallowing Disorders (Dysphagia)* (2012) 21:3-8.

Ashford J, McCabe D, Wheeler-Hegland K, Frymark T, Mullen R, Musson N, Schooling T, Smith Hammond C: Evidence-based systematic review: Oropharyngeal dysphagia behavioral treatments. Part III-Impact of dysphagia treatments on populations with neurological disorders. *Journal of Rehabilitation Research and Development* (2009) 46:195-204.

Ashford JR, Skelley M: Oral care and the elderly. *Perspectives on Swallowing and Swallowing Disorders (Dysphagia)* (2008) 17:19-26.

Bakhtiyari J, Sarraf P, Nakhostin-Ansari N, Tafakhori A, Logemann J, Faghihzadeh S, Harirchian MH: Effects of early intervention of swallowing therapy on recovery from dysphagia following stroke. *Iran J Neurol* (2015) 14:119-124.

Bakke M, Bardow A, Møller E: Severe Drooling and Treatment With Botulinum Toxin. *Perspectives on Swallowing and Swallowing Disorders (Dysphagia)* (2012) 21:15-21.

Barikroo A, Berretin-Felix G, Carnaby G, Crary M: Effect of transcutaneous electrical stimulation amplitude on timing of swallow pressure peaks between healthy young and older adults. *Gerodontology* (2015) DOI 10.1111/ger.12221.

Bedore B: Management of Dysphagia in Individuals with Amyotrophic Lateral Sclerosis. *Perspectives on Swallowing and Swallowing Disorders (Dysphagia)* (2013) 22:26-31.

Bours GH, *et al.*: Bedside Screening Tests Vs. Videofluoroscopy or Fiberoptic Endoscopic Evaluation of Swallowing to Detect Dysphagia in Patients with Neurological Disorders: Systematic Review. *Journal of Advanced Nursing* (2009) 65:477-93.

Brady L, Logemann J, Moss A: *ASHA Roundtable:* "What If a Patient Refuses Treatment?" (1997).

Butler SG, Pelletier CA, Steele CM: Compensatory Strategies and Techniques. In *Manual of Diagnostic and Therapeutic Techniques for Disorders of Deglutition.* Shaker R, Easterling, C, Belafsky PC, Postma GN (eds). Springer, New York, NY, 2012, pp. 299-316.

References

Carnaby G, Hankey GJ, Pizzi J: Behavioural intervention for dysphagia in acute stroke: A randomised controlled trial. *Lancet Neurology* (2006) 5:31-37.

Carnaby-Mann GD, Crary MA: Examining the evidence on neuromuscular electrical stimulation for swallowing. *Archives of Otolaryngology—Head and Neck Surgery* (2007) 133:564-71.

Carrau RL, Murry T: "Nonsurgical Treatment of Swallowing Disorders" (Chapters 34-37) and "Surgical Treatment of Swallowing Disorders" (Chapters 38-50) in *Comprehensive Management of Swallowing Disorders*, Carrau RL, Murry T (eds.), Singular Publishing Group, Inc. San Diego, CA, 1999, pp. 235-62, 263-343.

Carter J: Point/Counterpoint: Electrical Stimulation for Dysphagia: The Argument For Electrical Stimulation for Dysphagia. *Perspectives on Swallowing and Swallowing Disorders (Dysphagia)* (2011) 20:102-108.

Casarett D, Kapo J, Caplan A: Appropriate use of artificial nutrition and hydration—Fundamental principles and recommendations. *New England Journal of Medicine* (2005) 353:2607-12.

Chandran S: Surgical Management of Vocal Fold Paralysis and Cricopharyngeal Dysfunction as a Cause of Aspiration. *Perspectives on Swallowing and Swallowing Disorders (Dysphagia)* (2014) 23:106-115.

Ciucci MR, Grant LM, Rajamanickam ESP, Hilby BL, Blue KV, Jones CA, Kelm-Nelson CA: Early Identification and Treatment of Communication and Swallowing Deficits in Parkinson Disease. *Semin Speech Lang* (2013) 34:185-202.

Clark H, Lazarus C, Arvedson J, Schooling T, Frymark T: Evidence-based systematic review: Effect of neuromuscular electrical stimulation on swallowing and neural activation. *American Journal of Speech-Language Pathology* (2009) 18:361-75.

Coyle JL: Water, Water Everywhere, But Why? Argument Against Free Water Protocols. *Perspectives on Swallowing and Swallowing Disorders (Dysphagia)* (2011) 20:109-115.

Doidge N. *The Brain's Way of Healing. Remarkable Discoveries and Recoveries from the Frontiers of Neuroplasticity.* Viking, 2015.

Easterling C: Shaker Exercise. In *Manual of Diagnostic and Therapeutic Techniques for Disorders of Deglutition.* Shaker R, Easterling, C, Belafsky PC, Postma GN (eds). Springer, New York, NY, 2012, pp. 257-68.

Ebihara S, Kohzuki M, Sumi Y, Ebihara T: Sensory Stimulation to Improve Swallowing Reflex and Prevent Aspiration Pneumonia in Elderly Dysphagic People. *Journal of Pharmacological Sciences* (2011) 115:99-104.

Gawande A: "The way we age now." In *Annals of Medicine: The New Yorker,* April 30, 2007.

Goldsmith T, Jacobson MC: Revisiting Swallowing Function Following Contemporary Surgical Interventions for Oral/Oropharyngeal Cancer: Key Underlying Issues. *Perspectives on Swallowing and Swallowing Disorders (Dysphagia)* (2015) 24:89-98.

Gomes CA Jr, Andriolo RB, Bennett C, Lustosa SA, Matos D, Waisberg DR, Waisberg J: Percutaneous endoscopic gastrostomy versus nasogastric tube feeding for adults with swallowing disturbances. *Cochrane Database of Systematic Reviews* (2015) DOI 10.1002/14651858.

Hamdy S, Rothwell JC, Aziz Q, Thompson DG: Organization and reorganization of human swallowing motor cortex: Implications for recovery after stroke. *Clinical Science* (2000) 98:151-57.

Hamdy S: Role of Neurostimulation and Neuroplasticity in the Rehabilitation of Dysphagia After Stroke. *Perspectives on Swallowing and Swallowing Disorders (Dysphagia)* (2010) 19:3-9.

Heo SY, Kim KM: Immediate effects of Kinesio Taping on the movement of the hyoid bone and epiglottis during swallowing by stroke patients with dysphagia. *J Phys Ther Sci* (2015) 27:3355-57.

Hind JA, Robbins JHA: Oropharyngeal Strengthening and Rehabilitation of Deglutitive Disorders. In *Manual of Diagnostic and Therapeutic Techniques for Disorders of Deglutition.* Shaker R, Easterling, C, Belafsky PC, Postma GN (eds). Springer, New York, NY, 2012, pp. 237-55.

Hinson D, Goldsmith AJ, Murray J: Dysphagia in Hospice Care: The Roles of Social Work and Speech-Language Pathologists. *Perspectives*

References

on Swallowing and Swallowing Disorders (Dysphagia) (2014) 23:173-186.

Hopper T, Douglas N, Khayum B: Direct and Indirect Interventions for Cognitive-Communication Disorders of Dementia. *Perspectives on Neurophysiology and Neurogenic Speech and Language Disorders* (2015) 25:142-157.

Huckabee M-L: Rethinking Rehab: Skill-Based Training for Swallowing Impairment. *Perspectives on Swallowing and Swallowing Disorders (Dysphagia)* (2014) 23:46-53.

Huckabee M-L, Macrae P: Effortful Swallow. In *Manual of Diagnostic and Therapeutic Techniques for Disorders of Deglutition*. Shaker R, Easterling, C, Belafsky PC, Postma GN (eds). Springer, New York, 2012, pp. 281-98.

Hughes T, Watts CR: The Effects of Two Resistive Exercises on Electrophysiological Measures of Submandibular Muscle Activity. *Arch Phys Med Rehabil*. Dec. 2, 2015.

Humbert IA: Point/Counterpoint: Electrical Stimulation for Dysphagia: The Argument Against Electrical Stimulation for Dysphagia. *Perspectives on Swallowing and Swallowing Disorders (Dysphagia)* (2011) 20:102-8.

Jackson LD, Little J, Kung E, Williams EM, Siemiatkowska K, Plowman S: Safe Medication Swallowing in Dysphagia: A Collaborative Improvement Project. *Healthcare Quarterly* (2008) 11:110-16.

Jones *et al.*: Interventions for dysphagia in long-term, progressive muscle disease. *Cochrane Database of Systematic Reviews* (2016), Issue 2.

Kessing BF, Bredenoord AJ, Smout AJ: The pathophysiology, diagnosis and treatment of excessive belching symptoms. *Am J Gastroenterol* (2014) 109:1196-203.

Kind A, Anderson P, Hind J, Robbins JA, Smith M: Omission of Dysphagia Therapies in Hospital Discharge Communications. *Dysphagia* (2011) 26:49-61.

Krival K: Dysphagia Services in Nursing Homes: An Opportunity for Improving Patient Outcomes Through Palliative Care. *Perspectives on Gerontology* (2013) 18:88-102.

Landes TL: Ethical issues involved in patients' rights to refuse artificially administered nutrition and hydration and implications for the speech-language pathologist. *Am J Speech-Language Pathology* (1999) 8:109-17.

Langmore SE: Why I Like the Free Water Protocol. *Perspectives on Swallowing and Swallowing Disorders (Dysphagia)* (2011) 20:116-120.

Leder SB: Comparing Simultaneous Clinical Swallow Evaluations and Fiberoptic Endoscopic Evaluations of Swallowing: Findings and Consequences. *Perspectives on Swallowing and Swallowing Disorders (Dysphagia)* (2015) 24:12-17.

Lee KL, Kim DY, Kim WH, Kim EJ, Lee WS, Hahn SJ, Kang MS, Ahn SY: The influence of sour taste on dysphagia in brain injury: blind study. *Ann Rehabil Med* (2012) 36:365-70.

Leslie P, Casper M: Ethical Challenges: Less About Moral Wrongdoing and More About Communication Breakdown. *Perspectives on Gerontology* (2015) 20:72-84.

Levine P: Neuroplastic Model for Dysphagia. *Advance for Speech and Hearing* (2009) 19:10.

Leyden JE, Moss AC, MacMathuna P: Endoscopic pneumatic dilation versus botulinum toxin injection in the management of primary achalasia (Review). *Cochrane Database of Systematic Reviews* (2014) DOI 10.1002/14651858.

Lieberman A, McCall M: *100 Questions & Answers About Parkinson Disease.* Jones and Bartlett Publishers, Sudbury, MA (2003) pp. 123-27, 158-61.

Logemann JA: "Management of the Patient with Oropharyngeal Swallowing Disorders" (pp. 191-250); "Multidisciplinary Management of Dysphagia"(pp. 367-73), in *Evaluation and Treatment of Swallowing Disorders, 2nd ed.*, PRO-ED, Inc., Austin, TX (1998).

Logemann JA: Oropharyngeal dysphagia and nutritional management. *Current Opinion in Clinical Nutrition and Metabolic Care* (2007) 10:611-14.

Logemann JA: Debates in Dysphagia Management: How Do You Use Evidence-Based Practice in Your Dysphagia Patient Care?

References

Perspectives on Swallowing and Swallowing Disorders (Dysphagia) (2011) 20:121-123.

Logemann JA, Curro FA, Pauloski B, Gensler G: Aging effects on oropharyngeal swallow and the role of dental care in oropharyngeal dysphagia. *Oral Dis* (2013) 19:733-37.

Logemann JA *et al.*: A randomized study of three interventions for aspiration of thin liquids in patients with dementia or Parkinson's disease. *Journal of Speech, Language, and Hearing Research* (2008) 51:173-83.

Logemann J, Sonies B: "Grand rounds: Dysphagia." *The ASHA Leader*, July 20, 2004.

Ludlow C: Electrical stimulation and dysphagia: What we do and don't know. *The ASHA Leader*, March 4, 2008.

Lundy D, Sullivan P: Xerostomia. *Perspectives on Swallowing and Swallowing Disorders (Dysphagia)* (2012) 21:22-27.

Macrae P, Anderson C, Humbert I: Mechanisms of Airway Protection During Chin-Down Swallowing. *Journal of Speech, Language, and Hearing Research* (2014) 57:1251-58.

Malandraki GA, Johnson S, Robbins JA: Functional Magnetic Resonance Imaging of Swallowing Function: From Neurophysiology to Neuroplasticity. Published online September 7, 2011. Final edited form: *Head Neck* (2011) 33:S14-20.

Mason-Baughman MB, Kinder R: Dementia Management: A Practice Update for Speech-Language Pathologists. *Perspectives on Neurophysiology and Neurogenic Speech and Language Disorders* (2015) 25:158-164.

McColloch NL, Carroll WR, Magnuson JS: Pretreatment Dysphagia Protocol for the Patient with Head and Neck Cancer Undergoing Chemoradiation. *Perspectives on Swallowing and Swallowing Disorders (Dysphagia)* (2010) 19:53-56.

Medina-Walpole AM, Katz PR: Nursing home-acquired pneumonia. *Journal of the American Geriatrics Society* (1999) 47:1005-15.

Meier A: Lingual Strengthening: Success in an Outpatient Setting. *Perspectives on Swallowing and Swallowing Disorders (Dysphagia)* (2015) 24:71-74.

Melina A, Forest J: *Cooking Vegan: Healthful, Delicious, and Easy.* Book Publishing Company, Summertown, TN, 2012.

Miao M, Power E, O'Halloran R: Factors affecting speech pathologists' implementation of stroke management guidelines: a thematic analysis. *Disability and Rehabilitation* (2015) 37:674-85.

Miller AJ: Neuroscience of swallowing: Strategies in rehabilitation. *Perspectives on Swallowing and Swallowing Disorders (Dysphagia)* (2008) 17:121-27.

Mitchell SL: A 93-year-old man with advanced dementia and eating problems. *JAMA* (2007) 298:2527-36.

Mojon P: Oral health and respiratory infection. *Journal of the Canadian Dental Association* (2002) 68:340-05.

Morrison RS, Meier DE: Palliative care. *New England Journal of Medicine* (2004) 350:2582-90.

Mueller PS, Hook CC, Fleming KC: Ethical issues in geriatrics: A guide for clinicians. *Mayo Clinic Proceedings* (2004) 79:554-62.

National Institute on Aging: "Alzheimer's Disease and end-of-life issues." (2003) Last updated Feb. 26, 2015.

Nekl CG, Lintzenich CR, Leng X, Lever T, Butler SG: Effects of effortful swallow on esophageal function in healthy adults. *Neurogastroenterol Motil* (2012) 24:252-58.

Niedert KC, Dorner B (eds.): "Neurological Diseases" (pp. 80-84), "Dementia" (pp. 85-88), "Oral Health" (pp. 94-99), in *Nutrition Care of the Older Adult, 2nd ed.*, American Dietetic Association, Chicago, IL (2004).

Nund R, Ward E, Scarinci N, Cartmill B: The value of Qualitative Research in Dysphagia in the Head and Neck and Population: What Can We Learn From the Survivors' Perspective? *Perspectives on Swallowing and Swallowing Disorders (Dysphagia)* (2015) 24:99-106.

Ostwald SK, Davis S, Hersch G, Kelley C, Godwin KM: Evidence-based educational guidelines for stroke survivors after discharge home. *Journal of Neuroscience Nursing* (2008) 40:173-91.

Palmer JL, Metheny NA: Preventing aspiration in older adults with dysphagia. *Am J Nursing* (2008) 108:40-48.

References

Puntil-Sheltman J: Clinical Decisions Regarding Patients with Dysphagia and Palliative Care. *Perspectives on Swallowing and Swallowing Disorders (Dysphagia)* (2013) 22:118-123.

Riquelme LF: Managing Dysphagia in Long-Term Care Settings: Clinical Considerations. *Perspectives on Swallowing and Swallowing Disorders (Dysphagia)* (2013) 22:107-17.

Robbins J, Kays SA, Gangnon RE, Hind JA, Hewitt AL, Gentry LR, Taylor AJ: The effects of lingual exercise in stroke patients with dysphagia. *Archives of Physical Medicine and Rehabilitation* (2007) 88:150-58.

Robbins JA, Butler SG, Daniels SK, Gross RD, Langmore S, Lazarus CL, Martin-Harris B, McCabe D, Musson N, Rosenbek JC: Swallowing and Dysphagia Rehabilitation: Translating Principles of Neural Plasticity Into Clinically Oriented Evidence. *Journal of Speech, Language, and Hearing Research* (2008) 51:S276-300.

Robbins J, Hind JH: Swallow Stronger and Safer: Past, Present, and Future of the SwallowSTRONG Device. *Perspectives on Swallowing and Swallowing Disorders (Dysphagia)* (2015) 24:65-70.

Rogus-Pulia N, Hind J: Patient-Centered Dysphagia Therapy – The Critical Impact of Self-Efficacy. *Perspectives on Swallowing and Swallowing Disorders (Dysphagia)* (2015) 24:146-154.

Rosenbek J: Tactile-Thermal Stimulation in the Treatment of Dysphagia: Does It Have a Future? *Perspectives on Swallowing and Swallowing Disorders (Dysphagia)* (2014) 23:11-14.

Sapienza C, Wheeler-Hegland K, Stewart K, Nocera J: Exercise Prescription for Dysphagia: Intensity and Duration Manipulation. *Perspectives on Swallowing and Swallowing Disorders (Dysphagia)* (2008) 17:50-58.

Schneider SL, Haack L, Owens J, Herrington DP, Zelek A: An Interdisciplinary Treatment Approach for Soldiers with TBI/PTSD: Issues and Outcomes. *Perspectives on Neurophysiology and Neurogenic Speech and Language Disorders* (2009) 19:36-46.

Schwarz SP: Eating and drinking tips for people with swallowing difficulties. In Chapter 8 in *Parkinson's Disease: 300 Tips for Making Life Easier, 2nd ed.* Demos Medical Publishing, New York, NY, 2006, pp. 66-72.

Scutt P, Lee HS, Hamdy S, Bath PM: Pharyngeal Electrical Stimulation for Treatment of Poststroke Dysphagia: Individual Patient Data Meta-Analysis of Randomised Controlled Trials. *Stroke Res Treat* (2015) DOI 10.1155/2015/429053.

Shaker R, Antonik S: The Shaker exercise. *US Gastroenterology Review* (2006) 2:19-20.

Sharp HM, Bryant KN: Ethical issues in dysphagia: When patients refuse assessment or treatment. *Seminars in Speech and Language* (2003) 24:285-99.

Shastri N, Hogan W: Eosinophilic Esophagitis: The New Kid on the Block. *Perspectives on Swallowing and Swallowing Disorders (Dysphagia)* (2012) 21:43-51.

Smith Hammond CA, Goldstein LB: Cough and aspiration of food and liquids due to oral-pharyngeal dysphagia: ACCP evidence-based clinical practice guidelines. *Chest* (2006) 129:154S-168S.

Span P: *When the Time Comes: Families with Aging Parents Share their Struggles and Solutions.* Springboard Press, New York, NY (2006).

Stead A, McDonnell C: Discussing End of Life Care: An Opportunity. *Perspectives Geron* (2015) 20:12-15.

Stewart C: Dysphagia Symptoms and Treatment in Huntington's Disease: Review. *Perspectives on Swallowing and Swallowing Disorders (Dysphagia)* (2012) 21:126-134.

Sura L, Madhavan A, Carnaby G, Crary M: Dysphagia in the elderly: management and nutritional considerations. *Clinical Interventions in Aging* (2012) 7:287-98.

Tanner DC, Culbertson WF: Avoiding Negative Dysphagia Outcomes. *Onlin J Issues Nurs* (2014) Vol. 19, No. 2.

Troche MS: Respiratory Muscle Strength Training for the Management of Airway Protective Deficits. *Perspectives on Swallowing and Swallowing Disorders (Dysphagia)* (2015) 24:58-64.

Troche MS, Okun MS, Rosenbek JC, Musson N, Fernandez HH, Rodriguez R, Romrell J, Pitts T, Wheeler-Hegland KM, Sapienza CM: Aspiration and swallowing in Parkinson disease and rehabilitation with EMST: A randomized trial. *Neurology* (2010) 75:1912-19.

References

Troche MS, Rosenbek JC, Okun MS, Sapienza CM: Detraining outcomes with expiratory muscle strength training in Parkinson disease. *Journal of Rehabilitation Research and Development* (2014) 51:305-310.

Vollman J, Burke WJ, Kupfer RY, Tessler S, Friedel DM, Ozick LA, Gillick M: Rethinking the role of tube feeding in patients with advanced dementia. *New England Journal of Medicine* (2000) 342:206-10.

Voyzey G: Meeting the Cultural, Therapeutic, and Individual Needs of the Lesbian, Gay, Bisexual or Transgendered Patient. *Perspectives on Gerontology* (2014) 129:100-104.

Wallace G: Speech-Language Pathology: Enhancing Quality of Life for Individuals Approaching Death. *Perspectives on Gerontology* (2015) 20:85-103.

Wallace GL: Blast Injury Basics: A Primer for the Medical Speech-Language Pathologist. *The ASHA Leader* (2006) 11:26-28.

Waters SO, Sullivan PA: An Approach to Guiding and Supporting Decision-Making for Individuals with Dementia: Feeding, Swallowing, and Nutrition Considerations. *Perspectives on Swallowing and Swallowing Disorders (Dysphagia)* (2012) 21:105-111.

Weihoffen DL, Robbins J, Sullivan PA: *Easy-to-Swallow, Easy-to-Chew Cookbook. Over 150 Tasty and Nutritious Recipes for People Who Have Difficulty Swallowing.* John Wiley and Sons, NY, 2002.

Wheeler-Hegland K, Ashford J, Frymark T, McCabe D, Mullen R, Musson N, Smith Hammond C: Schooling T: Evidence-based systematic review: Oropharyngeal dysphagia behavioral treatments. Part II-Impact of dysphagia treatment on normal swallow function. *Journal of Rehabilitation Research and Development* (2009) 46:185-94.

Winchester J, Winchester CG: Cognitive Dysphagia and Effectively Managing the Five Systems. *Perspectives on Gerontology* (2015) 20:116-132.

Xie Y, Wang L, He J, Wu T: Acupuncture for dysphagia in acute stroke. *Cochrane Database Syst Rev* (2008) DOI 10.1002/14651858.

Yoon WL, Khoo JK, Rickard Liow SJ: Chin tuck against resistance (CTAR): New method for enhancing suprahyoid muscle activity using a Shaker-type exercise. *Dysphagia* (2014) 29:243-248.

Young CA, Ellis, Johnson J, Sathasivam S, Pih N: Treatment for sialorrhea (excessive saliva) in people with motor neuron disease/amyotrophic lateral sclerosis (Review). *Cochrane Database of Systematic Reviews* (2011) DOI 10.1002/14651858.

Chapter 9. Mindful Swallow, Safe Swallow

Bays JC: *Mindful Eating: A Guide to Rediscovering a Healthy and Joyful Relationship with Food.* Shambhala Press, Boston, MA, 2009.

Greger M, Stone G: *How Not To Die.* Flatiron Books, New York, NY, 2015.

Kabat-Zinn J: *Mindfulness for Beginners: Reclaiming the Present Moment and Your Life.* Sounds True, Louisville, CO, 2012.

Robbins J: *Diet for a New America: How Your Food Choices Affect Your Health, Happiness and the Future of Life on Earth, 2nd ed..* HJ Kramer/New World Library, Novato, CA, 2012.

Somov, PG: *Eating the Moment: 141 Mindful Practices To Overcome Overeating One Meal at a Time.* New Harbinger Publications, Oakland, CA, 2008.

ADDITIONAL READINGS

Avadian B: *"Where's My Shoes?" My Father's Walk Through Alzheimer's, 2nd ed.* North Star Books, Pearblossom, CA, 2005.

Bursack, CB: *Minding Our Elders. Caregivers Share Their Personal Stories.* McCleery & Sons, Publishing, Fargo, ND, 2005.

Campbell TC, Jacobson H: *Whole: Rethinking the Science of Nutrition.* BenBella Books, Dallas, TX, 2014.

Coskie, DF-S: *Unthinkable: Tips for Surviving a Child's Traumatic Brain Injury.* A Caregiver's Companion. Wyatt-MacKenzie Publishing, Deadwood, OR, 2011.

Davis B, Melina V: *Becoming Vegan: The Complete Reference To Plant-Based Nutrition.* Book Publishing Co., Summertown, TN, 2014.

Doidge N. *The Brain That Changes Itself: Stories of Personal Triumph from the Frontiers of Brain Science.* James H. Silberman Books, New York, NY, 2007.

Gawande A: *Being Mortal: Medicine and What Matters in the End*, Metropolitan Books, New York, NY, 2014.

Mace N, Rabins P: *The 36-Hour Day: A Family Guide to Caring for People with Alzheimer Disease, Related Dementias, and Memory Loss, 5th ed.* Hachette Book Group, New York, NY, 2012.

Marcell J: *Elder Rage—or, Take My Father...Please!* Impressive Press, Irvine, CA, 2001.

Martensen R: *A Life Worth Living: A Doctor's Reflections on Illness in a High-Tech Era*. Farrar, Strauss and Giroux, New York, NY, 2008.

McCullough D: *My Mother, Your Mother: Embracing "Slow Medicine" – The Compassionate Approach to Caring For Your Aging Loved Ones*. HarperCollins Publishers, New York, NY, 2008.

Mitra S, Ludka T, Rezkalla SH, Sharma PP, Luo J: Swallow Syncope: A Case Report and Review of the Literature. *Clin Med Res* (2011) 9:125-29.

New York Times: "At 96, Dr. Heimlich Uses His Own Maneuver on Choking Victim." May 27, 2016.

Northrup C: *Mother-Daughter Wisdom: Understanding the Crucial Link Between Mothers, Daughters, and Health*. Random House Publishing Group, New York, NY, 2006.

Sapienza C, Troche M, Pitts T, Davenport P: Respiratory muscle strength training [RMST]: concept and intervention outcomes. *Semin Speech Lang* (2011) 32:21-30.

Seuss D: *You're Only Old Once!* Random House, Inc., New York, NY, 1986.

Span P: *When the Time Comes: Families with Aging Parents Share Their Struggles and Solutions*. Springboard Press, New York, NY, 2009.

Winakur J: *Memory Lessons: A Doctor's Story*. Hyperion. New York, NY, 2009.

RESOURCES

Alzheimer Disease

Alzheimer's Association
www.alz.org
(800) 272-3900

Alzheimer's Disease
Education and Referral
Center (ADEAR), U.S.
NIH, National Institute
On Aging
https://www.nia.nih.gov/
alzheimers
(800) 438-4380

Alzheimer's Foundation
of America
www.alzfdn.org
(866) 232-8484

Alzheimer Society of
Canada
www.alzheimer.ca
(416) 488-8772

Blogs

The Caregiver's Voice
www.thecaregiversvoice.
com

The New Old Age:
Caring and Coping
New York Times
newoldage.blogs.
nytimes.com/

Transition Aging Parents
www.
transitionagingparents.
com/blog
(574) 261-8951

Caregiving

American Association of
Retired Persons (AARP)
www.aarp.org
(888) 687-2277

Caregiver.com
www.caregiver.com
(800) 829-2734

Caregiver Action Network
Cafregiveraction.org
(202) 454-3970

Eldercare Locator
www.eldercare.gov
(800) 677-1116

Family Caregiver Alliance
www.caregiver.org
(800) 445-8106

Leading Age
leadingage.com
(202) 783-2242

National Alliance
for Caregiving
www.caregiving.org
(301) 718-8444

National Council on Aging
www.ncoa.org
(571) 527-3900

Drug Information

FDA: United States
Food and Drug
Administration
www.fda.gov
(888) 463-6332

MedlinePlus
United States National
Library of Medicine
www.nlm.nih.gov/
medlineplus/

Legal

Justice in Aging
www.justiceinaging.org
(202) 289-6976

National Academy of
Elder Law Attorneys
www.naela.com

Multiple Sclerosis

Multiple Sclerosis
Association of America
www.msassociation.org
(800) 532-7667

National Multiple
Sclerosis Society
www.nationalmssociety.org
(800) 344-4867

Nutrition

Nutrition Facts
nutritionfacts.org
Michael Greger, M.D.
P.O. Box 11400
Takoma Park, MD 20913

T. Colin Campbell Center
for Nutrition Studies
nutritionstudies.org
P.O. Box 7256
Ithaca, NY 14851
(607) 319-0287

Parkinson Disease

American Parkinson
Disease Association
www.apdaparkinson.org
(800) 223-2732

Michael J. Fox Foundation
for Parkinson's Research
www.michaeljfox.org
(800) 708-7644

National Parkinson
Foundation
www.parkinson.org
(800) 473-4636

Parkinson's Disease
Foundation
www.pdf.org
(800) 457-6676

Stroke

American Stroke
Association
www.StrokeAssociation.org
(888) 478-7653

Heart and Stroke
Foundation of Canada
www.heartandstroke.com

National Institute of
Neurological Disorders
and Stroke
www.ninds.nih.gov

National Stroke Association
www.stroke.org
(800) 787-6537

Additional Resources

ALS Association
www.alsa.org
(800) 782-4747

American Autoimmune
Related Disease
Association
www.aarda.org
(586) 776-3900

American Board of
Swallowing
and Swallowing Disorders
www.swallowingdisorders.
org
(920) 560-5625

American Brain
Tumor Association
www.abta.org
(800) 886-2282

American Cancer Society
www.cancer.org
(800) 227-2345

American College of
Lifestyle Medicine
www.lifestylemedicine.org
(971) 983-5383

American Society on Aging
www.asaging.org
(800) 537-9728

American Speech-
Language-Hearing
Association (ASHA)
www.asha.org
(800) 638-8255

Cancer Care
www.cancercare.org
(800) 813-4673

Dysphagia Research Society
www.dysphagiaresearch.org
(713) 965-0566

Hastings Center
www.thehastingscenter.org
(845) 424-4040

Huntington's Disease
Society of America
www.hdsa.org
(800) 345-4372

Making Life Easier
www.makinglifeeasier.com
(608) 824-0401

Muscular Dystrophy
Association
www.mda.org
(800) 572-1717

Myasthenia Gravis
Foundation of America
www.myasthenia.org
(800) 541-5454

National Foundation
of Swallowing Disorders
www.swallowingdisorder
foundation.com
(415) 326-3673

National Hospice and
Palliative Care Organization
www.nhpco.org
(703) 837-1500

Oral Cancer Foundation
www.oralcancer.org
(949) 723-4400

Sri Sri Ravi Shankar
www.srisriravishankar.org
2401 15th St. NW
Washington, DC 20009

U.S. Administration
on Aging
www.aoa.gov

Wilson Disease
Association
www.wilsonsdisease.org
(866) 961-0533
(414) 961-0533

INDEX

Numbers in italics refer to
References, Additional Readings and **Resources**

A

abdominal thrusts. *See*
  Heimlich maneuver
acetylcholine, 79, 80
achalasia, 44, 132, *185*
acupuncture, *190*
advance directive, 134, 137
aging, effects of, 32, 43, *169*,
  170, *174*, *182*, *185*, *187*,
  189, *194*
alcohol, 32, 36, 69, 73, 145
ALS. *See* amyotrophic lateral
  sclerosis
Alzheimer disease, 6, 7, 33,
  34, 68, *170*, *187*, *193*,
  195. *See also*
  dementia
amyotrophic lateral sclerosis,
  6, 10, 31, 34, 37, 39, 66,
  100, 129, 132, *167*, *181*,
  190-91, *197*
  silent aspiration and, 68
anticholinergic drugs, 81, 82,
  83, 87, 101, 133, 161-63,
  175, *177*
  definition of, 79

listed, 82, 161-63
side effects, 79-83
therapeutic effects, 80
anxiety, 9, 29, 36, 47, 78, 84,
  91, 94, 101, 126, 137
  choking and, 47
  mouth-breathing and, 36
  pill-taking, 78, 91
ASHA (American Speech-
  Language-
  Hearing Association), 99,
  167, *172*, *177*, *180*, *181*,
  185, *186*, *190*, *197*
aspiration, 4, 8, 18, 29, 30, 36,
  37, 39, 40, 42, 43, 57, 61,
  65-73, 104, 106, 107, 108,
  110, 115, 118, 120-126,
  128, 130, 132, 135, 136,
  139, 144, *169*, *170*, *171*,
  172, *173*, *174*, *175*, *189*
  causes of, 36, 39, 40, 42, 43,
  67, 69, 80, 100, 118, 120
  chest x-rays and, 106-07
  deaths due to, 4
  definition, 65
  foods of mixed
  consistency and, 118-19

Index